# Vine OF THE Soul

## Medicine Men, their Plants and Rituals in the Colombian Amazonia

Richard Evans Schultes, F.M.L.S.
Robert F. Raffauf, F.L.S.

Foreword by Ghillean T. Prance, F.L.S.
Director, Royal Botanic Garden, Kew

Epilogue by Michael J. Balick, F.L.S.
Director and Philecology Curator of Economic Botany,
Institute of Economic Botany, The New York Botanical Garden

SYNERGETIC
PRESS

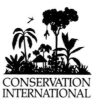

CONSERVATION
INTERNATIONAL

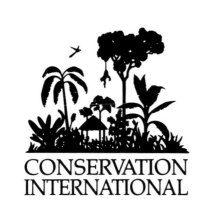

CONSERVATION
INTERNATIONAL

Synergetic Press is proud to support the efforts of Conservation International, a private, nonprofit organization dedicated to the conservation of tropical and temperate ecosystems worldwide. A percentage of the sale of this book goes to support Conservation International.

Published by
Synergetic Press, Inc.
Post Office Box 689
Oracle, Arizona 85623

ISBN 0 907791 24 7

Book designed by Debra K. Niwa, Design Distinction, Tucson, Arizona
Printed in the United States of America by Arizona Lithographers, Tucson, Arizona.

Printed on recycled paper.

# Contents

# Dedication

It is both a pleasure and an honour to dedicate this volume to
our friend,

Professor Gerardo Reichel-Dolmatoff Sci. D., F.L.S.,

celebrated field anthropologist, perceptive interdisciplinary scientist, prolific author, dedicated conservationist and understanding friend of the Indians and their culture. His research has been
a major factor in the enactment of wise laws by the Republic of
Colombia towards protection of its indigenous peoples.

Our lips shall tell them to our sons,
And they again to theirs ....
That generations yet unborne.
May teach them to their heirs.

Isaac Watts (1674-1748)

# Foreword

Professor Richard Evans Schultes and Professor Robert F. Raffauf have offered us an exciting new book which will help elucidate the need for one aspect of conservation—ethnobotanical conservation of a rich heritage which is in great danger of disappearing forever.

Schultes, the father of contemporary ethnobotany, is making prolific use of his retirement to present the results of his lifelong study of Amazon Indians. It is good to welcome his second book with Synergetic Press in its enjoyable format. During his field work, in addition to collecting plant specimens and ethnobotanical information, Schultes amassed a large collection of black-and-white photographs taken between 1941-1961, before the advent of modern automated cameras. They are a remarkable record of Indian life. Just keeping a camera functioning in the humid environment of Amazonia is an achievement, but these are exceptional views of various aspects of life of the tribes of the Colombian Amazonia. The importance of this record cannot be overemphasised, because these images were taken while Amazonia remained relatively pristine, and the tribes lived little touched by the influence of Western Civilization.

Although some acculturation of the people has since taken place, the Colombian Amazonia is where the future of tribal peoples has the most hope. Thanks to the attention drawn to the Indians by Schultes and his Colombian colleagues, the former President of Colombia, Virgilio Barco, returned to the Indians ownership of 6,000,000 hectares of the Colombian Amazon. In the ceremony in La Chorrera, country of the Witotos of the Colombian Amazonia, President Barco said in April 1988: "I have come to give you some good news, a word of truth; at last, the land which is yours *is* yours". In addition, a number of biological reserves have been made in the Colombian Amazon by the government, bringing the total area under protection to more than 20,000,000 hectares, an area slightly smaller than the United Kingdom. It is to be hoped that this example will be followed by other Amazonian nations. Where these Indians live, the forest is not destroyed and thus the Indians likewise conserve the species-rich rain forest of the northwest Amazon. The most efficient way to conserve rain forests is to have them cared for by natives, who will use them with little or no destruction of the ecosystem.

The aspect of Indian life which forms the focus of this book is the native's use of hallucinogenic and other sacred plant drugs. This study has long been the specialty of Professor Schultes and many of his students. The use of these plants and the associated rituals is central to Indian life. The extent to which the Indians have discovered so many species with active chemical compounds from such a rich array of the plant kingdom is remarkable. Their use has certainly inspired medicine men (or payés, as they are better called in this book) to find new medicines. This route has been one of the most important ways by which new medical agents have been discovered. Today, as pharmaceutical companies search for new plant-based medicines, undoubtedly some of them will come from the knowledge possessed by Amazonian payés.

Although this book is primarily a photographic essay, it contains a wealth of ethnobotanical information, distilled from a long

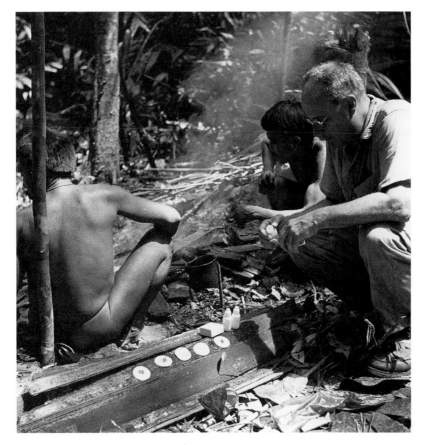

*In many cases, it is possible to test freshly collected plants in the field for the types of chemical compounds which may be responsible for their medicinal or toxic use.*

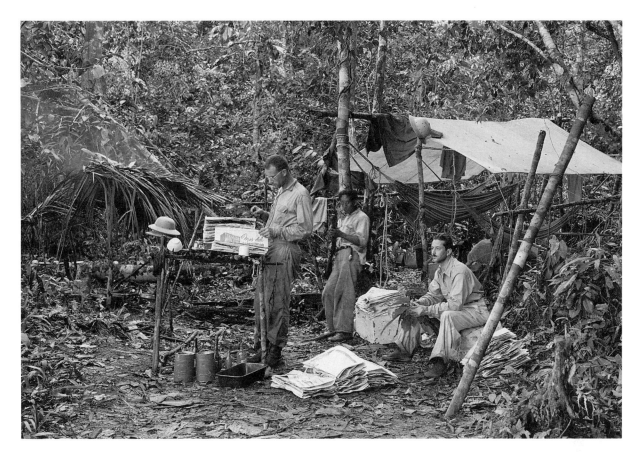

*The collection of voucher herbarium specimens is essential for exact identification of plants on which reports of use are based. These specimens, either dried in the field or preserved in formaldehyde for later drying, are prepared usually when the reports are given.*

series of scientific papers by Schultes and his many students. Thus we have accurate scientific data presented in a readily understandable format. Since the second author, Raffauf, is an outstanding plant chemist who has devoted most of his research to the elucidation of the chemical structure of bioactive compounds in plants, this volume contains also much up-to-date chemical information.

We have here a wonderful integration of ethnobotany, chemistry and photography to produce a book that will long be an important historic record of one of the threatened cultures of the world. I hope that readers learning about ayahuasca, the vine of the soul, and the other psychoactive drugs discussed here will have their concern heightened for the future fate of Amazon Indians and their societies.

Ghillean T. Prance, F.L.S.
Director, Royal Botanic Garden, Kew

# Introduction

We have chosen as the title of our book a translation of the Ketchwa word ayahuasca, a widely employed name used by numerous Indian tribes of Peru, Ecuador and Colombia for the hallucinogenic liana *Banisteriopsis Caapi*, the most important of the many sacred plants in the repertoire of the shamans throughout the western Amazonia.

Specialists amongst the ethnologists and anthropologists may object on the ground that many of the tribes of the Colombian Amazonia with which this book is concerned do not have the concept of "soul" as it is generally understood and that terms such as *vine of vision, vine of insight, vine of wisdom* or *vine of enlightenment*, for example, might be more appropriate. There are numerous other Indian names for the plant: *yajé*, used in the southern parts of the Colombian Amazonia, and *caapi*, employed in the Vaupés of Colombia and adjacent Brazil, are two common terms.

Yet none of these, in our opinion, convey to the general reader the importance of this vine to Indian culture. They do not so effectively describe the other-worldly experiences in which these Indians believe they can communicate through visual and auditory hallucinations with the supernatural world, the spirits of the ancestors, the plants, animals and the mythological beings of this vast region as does "vine of the soul".

This book is the story of a time that was—a time when the Amazon Indian was free to roam the forests and the rivers, happy with the social institutions that he had developed, unencumbered by acculturation, the cultural destruction of his ancient societies and his virgin forests brought about by the intrusion of commercial interests, missionary efforts, tourism and supposedly well-intentioned governmental or bureaucratic attempts to replace this precious heritage of an aboriginal people with something alien to their culture and its natural environment. We have chosen to tell the story in a series of photographs taken during field expeditions over the last 45 years. For each illustration we have selected an appropriate quotation taken from the writings of the early explorers, botanists, anthropologists and others who have devoted much of their lives to the study of the Amazon and its people and the apparently odd customs, superstitions, religious beliefs and rituals practiced by these indigenous groups whose ancestors came to the region during the Amerindian migrations at least 25,000 years ago.

Amongst the earliest of human experiences was the discovery that some plants could serve as sources of food and shelter, while others, when eaten or rubbed on the skin, relieved distress, eased pain and made life more tolerable in other ways. Certainly, some of the unworldly effects, such as those produced by the hallucinogens, must have been startling. It is no wonder, then, that the knowledge and use of the properties and uses of these plants became identified with certain individuals in the community, the *shaman* or *medicine man*. And in view of primitive beliefs in a spirit world which controls the destinies of mankind, it is understandable that magical or supernatural properties were ascribed to certain plants and that some of them were even considered sacred because of their extraordinary psychoactivity through which this individual believed that he would be able, during his trances, to visit the realms of the spirit.

This turn of events must certainly have been true of the very early Indians of the Americas, if we are to judge from archaeological remains and other evidence of the use of psychoactive plants. The power of the individual which is believed to reside in the knowledge and use of these plants is apparently stronger in South America than in any other part of the western hemisphere. And it is likely that the shaman's influence in the northwest Amazonia is more powerful and penetrating in all aspects of profane and magico-religious life than in other parts of the Amazon basin itself.

Several titles have been bestowed upon these specialized men or women. *Medicine man*, whilst usually all-inclusive and generally understood, may perhaps exclude some very successful practitioners who rarely, if ever, use medicinal plants. Although it is commonly employed in anthropological writings, the term *shaman*, of Asiatic origin, seems foreign to us in a New World context. The term *witch doctor*, which certainly describes many of the functions of these practitioners, we find unacceptable for its potential pejorative connotations. The designation *payé* is widely employed in most parts of the Amazon, and we tend to favour its use in our writing.

Our story focuses, then, on the payé, whose exalted place in the community depends on his knowledge of plants, respect or fear of his powers by his people and control of virtually all aspects of life by the use of these plants in well-established magico-religious, superstitious, ritualistic or ceremonial beliefs and practices.

Not all payés are medicine men, but most of them do have a rather extensive interest in the properties of plants and will resort to prescribing them when their superstitious diagnoses or treatments fail. When they want to commune with the supernatural world, they almost always resort to plants, usually the hallucinogens. Several of these are used: various species of *Brugmansia*; intoxicating snuff or pills made from the exudate from the inner bark of sundry species of *Virola*; or primarily the vision-inducing yajé, *Banisteriopsis Caapi*. Through use of this "vine of the soul", the payé believes he can diagnose and treat illnesses, prophesy and carry out his other numerous duties. With these religious and superstitious foundations, he is thought to be able to regulate birth and death; the choice of site, architecture and building of *malocas*; hunting and fishing; the weather; travel on the rivers and trips through the forests; the consecration of foods; agriculture, especially the growing of coca, tobacco and medicinal, toxic and hallucinogenic plants; the rearing of children; the construction of canoes; the preparation of curare and hallucinogenic drinks; along with countless other responsibilities.

Amongst the indigenous peoples of the Colombian Amazonia, and probably in primitive societies of the tropics in many regions, there are two general classes of plant medicines: those that are regarded as sacred and used exclusively by or under the strict surveillance of the payé, primarily the hallucinogens; and those known and used by the general population, often but not always known and collected by the women. Our research has included data from both sources—from the payés and from the general population.

It has rightly been stated that the payé and his authority are the "cultural cornerstones" of aboriginal life in the northwest Amazonia. This was recognized over a century and a half ago by scientists whose excursions into the Amazon laid the foundation for many of the subsequent studies of its people. In any review of ethnobotanical aspects of life amongst the Indians of the region, it seems appropriate to mention three of these astute observers whose writings sparkle with references to Indian uses and names of plants, their payés, their mythology, their superstitions and other aspects of aboriginal life. We do this, however, without depreciating the efforts of those who followed in their footsteps. Two of these pioneers were botanists, Karl F.P. von Martius and Richard Spruce; the third was an anthropologist, Theodor Koch-Grünberg.

Karl Friedrich Philipp von Martius (1794-1868) was an outstanding German plant explorer who, in 1820, was the first botanist-ethnobotanist to work in the Colombian Amazonia. He spent three years, from 1817 to 1820, almost always in Brazil, collecting plants from Río de Janeiro up to Belém do Pará. He then proceeded up the Río Amazonas and ascended into Colombian territory on the Río Caquetá as far west as the impassable rapids at Araracuara.

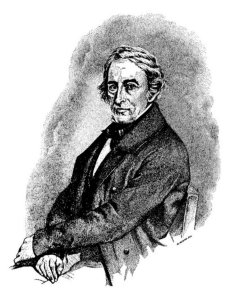

*K. F. P. von Martius, the first botanist to penetrate the Colombian Amazonia in 1820.*

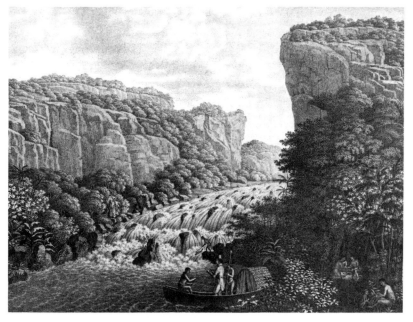

*The Falls of Araracuara on the Río Caquetá of Colombia, the farthest west that von Martius could penetrate in 1820. From Flora Brasiliensis*

He was a tireless collector, and his notes are rich in ethnobotanical observations and data on the numerous Indian tribes and their customs. His first published report, written jointly with the German zoologist Johann Baptist von Spix, *Reise in Brasilien*, was published in three volumes from 1824 to 1845. His greatest work, still consulted daily by botanists working on South American plants, was the monumental *Flora Brasiliensis*, which he founded in 1829. This encyclopedic compendium continued long after his death, until 1906, and throughout its entire preparation, it represented a collaboration of botanical specialists of many countries, a characteristic of von Martius' well known international outlook.

Richard Spruce (1817-1893), British born and botanically self-educated, was one of the greatest plant explorers of all times. He spent 15 years in South America, amassing a vast collection of plants, mostly trees, although his specialty was the bryophytes. From 1849 to 1855, he worked in the Brazilian Amazon and the upper Orinoco of Venezuela. From 1855 to 1864, his field of activity took him up the Amazon River and its Ecuadorian tributaries to the high Andes. Although he never worked in Colombia, he did collect amongst the Indians along its frontier with Brazil and Venezuela.

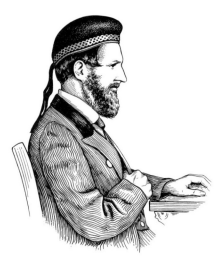

A man of limited means, he financed his field work by selling his specimens through Kew Gardens. His studies of *Hevea*, the genus of the rubber tree, and of *Cinchona*, source of quinine, have benefitted mankind and helped enrich governments and plantation industries. Spruce's field notes are replete with ethnobotanical notes, and one of his greatest discoveries was the identification of the "vine of the soul", *Banisteriopsis Caapi*.

The simplicity characteristic of his life and philosophy is the keynote on his gravestone in the churchyard of Terrington, Yorkshire: "Richard Spruce, traveller and author of many botanical books".

*A drawing of Richard Spruce from a photograph taken shortly before his departure for South America. Drawn by E. W. Smith, from a photograph in the Gray Herbarium.*

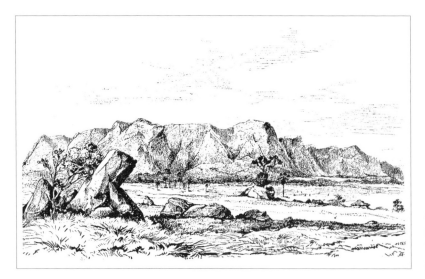

*A sketch of the Cerro Duida made by Richard Spruce from the Village of Esmeraldas on the upper Río Orinoco.*

Theodor Koch-Grünberg (1872-1924), German ethnologist and geographical explorer, was one of the greatest scientists to have worked in the northwest Amazonia and upper Orinoquia. His voluminous notes are available to us through his many articles and several books.

Between 1903 and 1905, he lived amongst the natives in the upper Río Negro basin of Brazil and in the Colombian Amazonia. The results of this stay are published in his two-volume *Zwei Jahre unter den Indianern* and stand today as the most comprehensive study of the cultures of that region; they have a wealth of ethnobotanical information.

From 1911 to 1913, he carried out an incredibly difficult journey from Mt. Roraima, which he climbed, across northernmost Brazil and southern Venezuela, mapping many unknown rivers and even making motion pictures of tribal ceremonies. This great achievement is outlined in his book *Von Roraima zum Orinoco*.

*Theodor Koch-Grünberg with Makuna Indians on the Río Apaporis.*

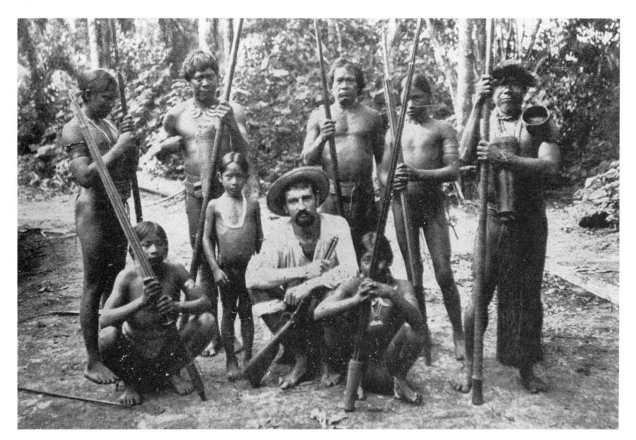

The scientific results of these two expeditions place Koch-Grünberg amongst those earlier Victorian naturalists whose interests and accomplishments were all-inclusive. He made anthropological, botanical and geological collections; more than 1000 photographs; records of temperature and atmospheric pressure; detailed descriptions of Indian myths, legends, magico-religious beliefs; and studies of more than 20 languages. His work is the basis of all modern research centered in the region.

Always on friendly terms with the Indians, he was an unpretentious gentleman, described as a scholar of "patience, courage and understanding". He respected the natives and was quick to condemn mistreatment of these, his friends. On a return visit to the Vaupés, he wrote:

"Hardly five years have gone by since my last visit to the Caiarý-Uaupés. Whoever comes here now will no longer find the pleasant place I once knew. The pestilential stench of a pseudo-civilisation has fallen on the brown people who have no rights. Like a swarm of annihilating grasshoppers, the inhuman gang of rubber barons continue to press forward. The Colombians already have settled in at the mouth of the Kuduyarí and carry off my friends to the death-dealing rubber forests. Raw brutality, mistreatment and murder are the order of the day. On the lower Caiarý the Brazilians are no better. The Indians' villages are desolate, their homes have been reduced to ashes and their garden plots, deprived of hands to care for them, are taken over by the jungle.

"Thus a vigorous race, a people endowed with a magnificent gift of bright intellect and gentle disposition will be reduced to naught. Human material capable of development will be annihilated by the brutality of these modern barbarians of culture".

Koch-Grünberg was associated with the Museum für Länder- und Völkerkunde in Stuttgart and the University of Freiburg. He died of malaria at Vista Alegre, Brazil, whilst on an expedition to the Sierra Parima headed by the geographer Hamilton Rice. He is buried there in the Amazonia that he loved.

An understanding of the role of the payé as the intermediary between the spiritual life and the day-to-day existence of his people would not be complete without some reference to the environment in which he functions.

# The Amazonia

The Amazon basin—that area of South America to which all tributaries drain into the Río Amazonas—is as extensive as the entire United States. One fifth of the world's fresh water is Amazonian, and the flora is the most diverse on the globe. The river systems drain areas in six countries: Bolivia, Brazil, Colombia, Ecuador, Peru and a small part of Venezuela. The Amazonia is the home of several hundred tribes of Indian peoples.

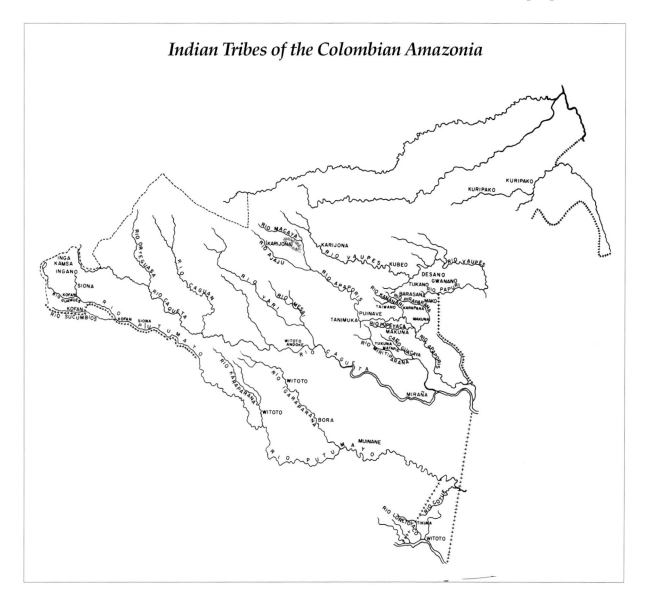

*Indian Tribes of the Colombian Amazonia*

# The Colombian Amazonia

While the Colombian Amazonia is, in reality, but a small sector of the whole basin, what is not well recognized is that nearly one third of the land surface of the Republic is Amazonian. This area is, in many respects, very different from the rest of the great basin. It is complex and varied, dropping from the eastern slopes of the Andes to the forested plains as low as 300 feet. The region is spotted with isolated quartzitic and, in the east, granitic moun-

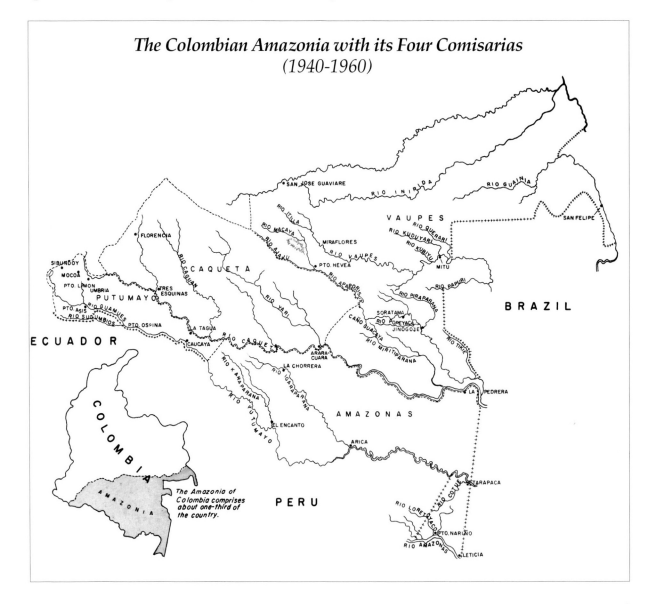

**The Colombian Amazonia with its Four Comisarias**
*(1940-1960)*

tains. All but one of Colombia's Amazonian rivers (the Putumayo) are not navigable because of interruptions by many rapids and waterfalls. And according to a recent census, the average density of population, mostly aboriginal, is approximately 0.33 inhabitants per square mile.

When most of the photographs in this book were taken (1941-1961), Amazonian Colombia comprised four *comisarías* or states: the Putumayo, Caquetá, Amazonas and Vaupés. Now it includes six, the largest, the Vaupés, having been reduced in size to create two additional divisions, the Guainía and the Guaviare. The four original comisarías, on which this book is based, make up a total of 155,800 square miles. There are few comparatively large centres of population: Sibundoy, Mocoa, Puerto Asís, Puerto Leguizamo, Leticia, Florencia, La Pedrera, Miraflores and Mitú.

The area is the home of a relatively large and very diverse Indian population. They speak many different languages and dialects. The Tukanoan family of languages is spoken in the Vaupés by Tukanos, Gwananos, Taiwanos, Kubeos, Karapanás, Desanos, Barasanas and Makunas, and in the west, the Sionas and Koreguajes. The Witotan family includes the language of the Witotos, Boras, Muinanes, Andokes, and Mirañas. In several other parts of the region, Indians speak languages belonging to the Arawakan family: the Yukunas, Tanimukas, Matapies, Kuripakos, Baniwas and possibly the Kawiyarís. The Tikunas of the Trapecio Amazónico are believed to speak an Arawakan language; the few remaining Karibs speak a Karib language. Numerous Puinaves have migrated into the Vaupés from the *llanos*, and they speak a language not yet classified. In Sibundoy, the Kamsás speak a language believed to be Chibchan; the Ingas of the Valley of Sibundoy and Mocoa speak an unmistakably Ketchwan language related to the speech of the ancient Incas. The Kofán language is tentatively related to the Chibchan family, but this is not a matter of general agreement. In the Vaupés, especially in the region of the Río Piraparaná, there are numerous groups of very primitive nomadic Makús; their language has still not been classified to any known family.

Degrees of acculturation vary and all are not of the same severity. Compared to many other parts of the Amazon, acculturation in the Colombian section has fortunately not been so extreme as in most other areas. A major reason is that Nature has protected the region with its waterfalls and rapids from intrusion from Brazil, and settlers from the malaria-free and fertile Andes have not been anxious to invade the Colombian Amazonia in great waves. Since the area is settled mostly by indigenous peoples, it has not suffered the extensive destruction of the forests which is typical of other Amazonian regions, especially that of Brazil. The Indian in Colombia, with his axe, fells only enough forest for his own agricultural needs. When these small clearings are eventually abandoned, the climax forest usually can recover and reestablish itself within 75 or 100 years. When, however, one million acres are mechanically felled and burned over to be used for only a few years for pasturage and then abandoned, as is common in Brazil, the climax forest will never recover, and the great area will forever be a scrub desert of weedy type growth.

From our point of view, there are many valuable and productive results to be expected from studies of the South American Indians and their ways of life. The anthropologist, the ethnologist, sociologist and psychologically trained specialists are naturally interested in the social aspects of ethnobotanical research and its relevance to their understanding of human life in general. Without attempting to intrude upon these fields of scientific enquiry, we must stress that our interest has been oriented towards the biological and pharmaco-chemical aspects, trying, at the same time, to appreciate and annotate the role of the payé in the medical, religious and superstitious facets of Indian life. It is, after all, impossible to separate the two spheres of interest when one is considering the knowledge of pre-literate societies. This viewpoint has been succinctly expressed by a celebrated anthropologist who writes: "One of the challenges facing ethnobotanists is to integrate the chemical, pharmacological and ecological study of plant-derived remedies into ethnomedical studies which focus on the social and symbolic functions of folk medicine" (Turner, in litt. 1990).

This task is not an easy one. There are an estimated 80,000 species of higher plants in the Amazonian flora. Recently, we published notes on some 1500 plants used as medicines or poisons in the northwest Amazonia alone; these species belong in 596 genera and 145 plant families (*The Healing Forest*, Dioscorides Press, 1990). They constitute those which are sacred and employed as hallucinogens by the payés but also those which are known to and used by the general population. Investigation into the vast array of chemical compounds produced by these plants in their extensive rain forest environment and which, in some instances, may have interesting and potential medical or industrial use has hardly begun. This heritage, amassed by aboriginal peoples over many hundreds of years and passed verbally from one generation to the next, is unfortunately fast disappearing as the result of acculturation and westernisation, or sadly, actual annihilation of the indigenous culture or even physical extinction of the tribe itself. In Colombia, the loss of this precious wealth of knowledge is not so prevalent: the government have created stringent laws and have set up a well planned programme of conservation of natural and ethnobotanical resources and protection of indigenous peoples which should, indeed, serve as a model for other Amazonian nations, if not for regions of tropical areas on other continents.

In presenting this photographic essay—in many ways a companion to an earlier volume**—we hope to offer a general overview, though certainly not a complete or technical one, of a complex topic that may not be widely understood and to help support Colombia's praiseworthy efforts to conserve tropical forests and the natives whose folklore we are but beginning to appreciate. It is also our hope to express the need for increasing programmes to include the recording of this ethnoscientific lore before it is forever entombed with the cultures that gave it birth. During our field work (one of us a botanist, the other a plant chemist), we found the Indians extremely friendly, cooperative and thoroughly in sympathy with our interest in their plant lore. Numerous payés collaborated willingly in our efforts, frequently accompanying us on our field trips. Without their help, our treks through the jungles and rivers would indeed have been more difficult and less productive.

**_Where the Gods Reign_, Richard Evans Schultes, Synergetic Press, 1988.

15

# Acknowledgements

Over the course of the numerous years of our research in the Colombian Amazonia, our results would have been appreciably diminished were it not for the generous assistance of many individuals and their organisations who made much of our work possible. We acknowledge with gratitude: The Indians of many tribes, their payés, herbalists and ordinary citizens who generously shared their knowledge of plants and their importance to the Indian way of life; the Institute of Natural Sciences of the National University of Colombia, for the physical support and the collaboration of the directors and scientific staff (Professors Alvaro Fernández-Pérez, Jesús Idrobo, Hernando García-Barriga, Luis Eduardo Mora, Roberto Jaramillo) and the technical staff (Mr. Mardoqueo Villarreal and his assistants) who cared for our specimens upon their arrival in Bogotá; the military and ecclesiastical personnel in the region; the several governors of the Amazonian comisarías or states; and the late Don Rafael Wandurraga of Leticia and Puerto Nariño whose dedication to and honourable treatment of the local Indians and his love for the forest and its preservation places him among the earliest and most effective conservationists of this part of Colombia.

Our gratitude must also be expressed to several of the government officials of the Repúblic, all of whom in recent years have been avid conservationists: especially former Presidents Dr. Misael Pastrana B., Dr. Belisario Betancur, and Dr. Virgilio Barco. We owe a debt for encouragement to Dr. Paulo Lugari, founder and director of the model agronomical and conservation station Las Gaviotas on the Río Vichada in the llanos of Colombia; his creative ideas of improving indigenous life in the tropics has had a potent and lasting influence on Colombian treatment of local peoples. We also recognise with appreciation the efforts in 1986 of Dr. Mariano Ospina H., then General Director of the Colombian Caja Agraria, who was instrumental in conceiving the Plan Integral del Predio Putumayo, a forward-looking programme beneficial to the Indians of the Colombian Amazon and their culture.

Knowledge often accumulates in small increments, and we express our debt to several pioneer anthropologists who worked in various parts of the Colombian Amazonia: Professor Gerardo Reichel-Dolmatoff, to whom this book is dedicated, Dr. and Mrs.

Stephen Hugh-Jones of Cambridge University, Dr. Martin von Hildebrand, founder of the experimental conservation settlement El Rastrojo on the lower Río Miritiparaná, and the late Dr. Peter Silverwood-Cope, whose research was carried out amongst the poorly known nomadic Makús of the Río Piraparaná.

Finally, we express our gratitude to several colleagues who have given us permission to include some of their outstanding photographs: the late Lothar Pedersen, M.D. (p. 70), the late Dr. Timothy Plowman (p. 45), Dr. James Zarucchi (pp. 109, 99), Prof. Hernando García-Barriga (p. 3), Dr. José Cuatrecasas (p. 64), Prof. Gerardo Reichel-Dolmatoff (p. 169), Dr. Jeffrey Hart (p. 63), and the Golden Press of New York for permission to reproduce two artistic illustrations prepared by the late Mr. Elmer W. Smith for their Golden Guidebook (Schultes: *Hallucinogenic Plants*) published in 1976 (pp. 173, 226). The crystals of scopolamine hydrobromide (p. 57) were isolated by one of the authors (R.F.R.).

We deeply appreciate the Danforth Conservation Biology Fund of the Roger Williams Park Zoo/Rhode Island Zoological Society, Conservation International, the World Wildlife Fund and Mr. Peter Thomson of Boston for financial assistance in the preparation of this book.

I have come to give you some good news, a word of truth: At last, the land which is yours *is* yours!

V. Barco (1988)
Former Colombian President

While the future payé is being initiated and invested with different powers, he and his master spend long hours singing and pronouncing incantations...

G. Reichel-Dolmatoff (1975)

The ability to cure sickness implies the ability to cause it. Shamans in tropical South American, with some exceptions, can always be sorcerers.

S.S. Robinson (1979)

Hardly any other [artistry] has called forth...so many varied and contradictory explanations as the [wall] drawings and figures...

T. Koch-Grünberg (1907)

For the American Indian, the presence in a plant of any psychotropic effect whatever was plain evidence of its containing supernatural "medicine" or spirit-shaking power.

W. La Barre (1972)

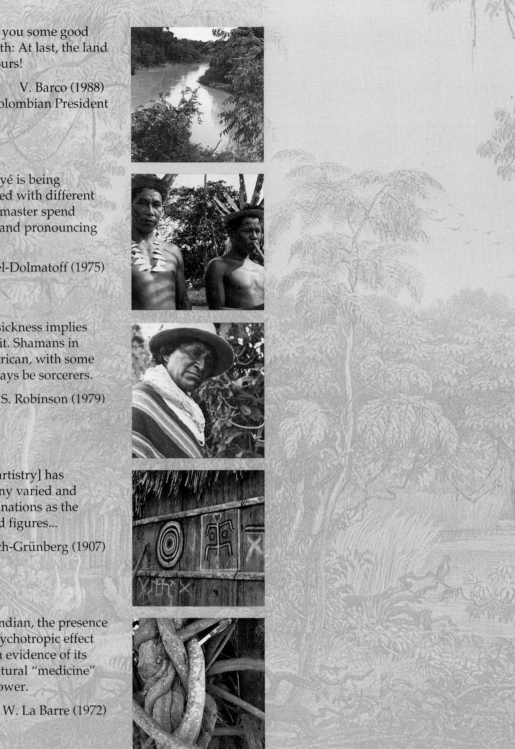

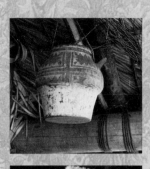

The characteristics which make the Indian love the ayahuasca beverage are, in addition to the visionary dreams, the pictures bearing on his personal happiness [and those in] which he sees..., beasts...demons...phantoms.

L. Lewin (1931)

The senses become extraordinarily acute and fine. The eyes pierce Infinity. The ear perceives the most imperceptible in the midst of the sharpest noises. Hallucinations begin. External objects take on monstrous appearances...sounds have odour and colours are musical.

C. Baudelaire (1860)

Herbalists avail themselves of the richness of the forest in a vast reservoir of medicinal ingredients capable of producing fragrant therapeutic odours ... [he] approaches a palm or tree not as an inert vegetable but as an anthropomorphic being.

J. Wilbert (1987)

Knowledge of how these species might prove useful for human welfare is often disappearing faster even than the tropical trees themselves, as the natives change their aboriginal life styles.

M.J. Plotkin (1981)

Who knows what plants of potential medical or other value, quite apart from their scientific interest, have already gone the way of the dodo?

R. Darnley Gibbs (1974)

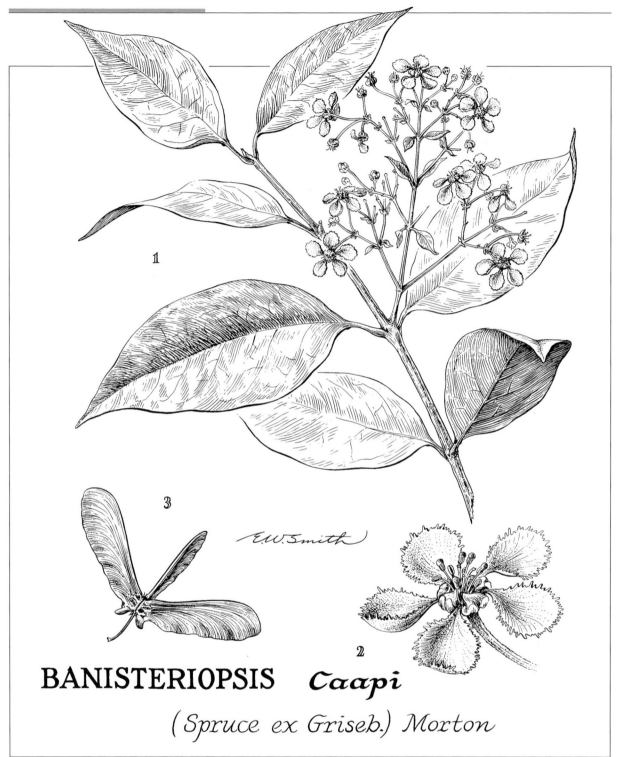

1

3

*E.W.Smith*

2

# BANISTERIOPSIS *Caapi*

## *(Spruce ex Griseb.) Morton*

…a man…(can) transfer the emotions…(and) intellect to unknown regions.

If human consciousness is the
most wonderful thing on earth,
the attempt to fathom the depths
of the psychophysiological action
of narcotic and stimulating drugs
makes this wonder seem greater
still, for with their help, man is
enabled to transfer the emotions
of everyday life, as well as his
intellect, to unknown regions.

L. Lewin (1931)

# The payé's most efficient tool

*Native throughout the western Amazonia*

Tukanoan imagery has a striking myth concerning caapi or yajé.
The river is a man with his feet at the river's mouth; his outspread
arms represent the affluents, and his head the source. The man is
shaking his flowing hair, out of which fall the leaves of a yajé vine.
They drop into the river, and even whilst falling they turn into
fish.

*Banisteriopsis Caapi* (of the Malpighiaceae or Malpighia Family)
has occupied the attention of scientists—botanists, anthropologists, chemist, pharmacologists, medical specialists—for more
than 50 years. A sacred hallucinogenic plant, it is nonetheless the
focal point of indigenous medical practise in the western
Amazonia.

The plant contains a group of alkaloids collectively known as *beta*-
carbolines of which harmine is the major component.

A shaman makes use of hallucinogens in order to obtain the visions which are his most important source of knowledge. "We drink yagé", says the payé..., "things begin to speak to us, and our souls are released from our bodies." In the *lingua geral* of the Vaupés, the most efficacious drug...is called yagé. The Quichua word is *ayahuasca*, which means "liana of the soul", while western scientists know it by the Latin name, *Banisteriopsis Caapi*.

F. Trupp (1981)

## Celebrated Makuna payé gathering "vine of the soul"

*Río Popeyaká, Amazonas*

Throughout the western Amazonia, a strongly intoxicating drink is made, the most widely employed hallucinogen of the region. In the westernmost Amazon of Colombia, the bark is scraped from a stout vine and boiled; in most of the Colombian Amazonia, the bark is simply kneaded in cold water. Occasionally, the resulting bitter drink is fortified with any of a number of other plants, some of which are themselves highly toxic. The two additives most frequently used are the leaves of *oco-yajé* or *chagropanga*, *Diplopterys Cabrerana* (Malpighiaceae) and *chacruna*, *Psychotria viridis* (Rubiaceae).

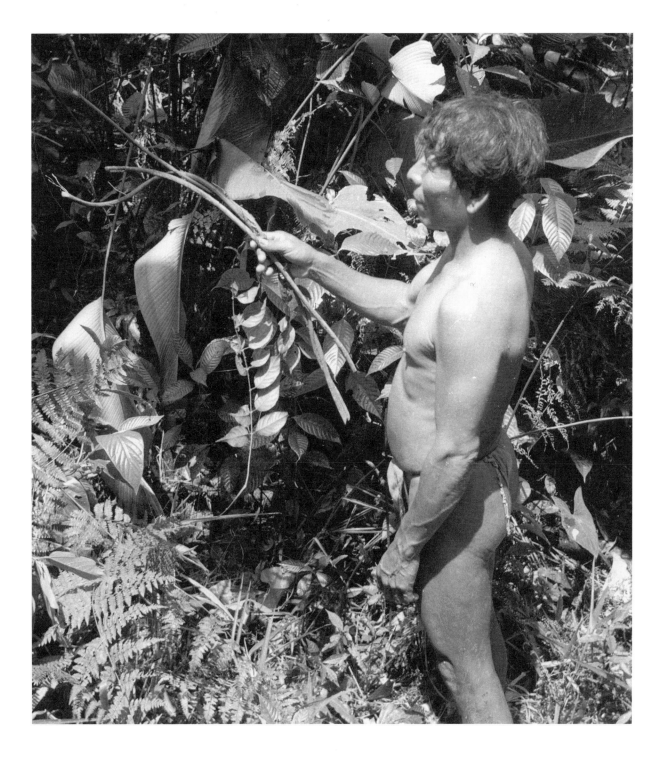

Liana of the soul..., *Banisteriopsis Caapi*.

Yajé is grown from cuttings
and is thus thought to be one
continuous vine which stretches
back to the beginning of time....
yajé itself is compared to an
umbilical cord that links human
beings...to the mythical past.

S. Hugh-Jones (1979)

# Cultivation of the "vine of the soul" in a Makuna garden

*Río Piraparaná, Vaupés*

The medicine men prefer to make their intoxicating caapi drink from old lianas growing in the jungle. These, however, are getting scarce, and many of the practitioners cultivate the plant in their coca gardens. It is not difficult to cultivate from cuttings. The psychic effects of the "vine of the soul" differ sometimes strikingly, according to the environmental and ceremonial background against which it is taken; the additives, if any, that are used in its preparation, the amount of the drug imbibed, the strength of auto-suggestion on the part of the Indian and numerous other factors.

There are, however, certain effects which seem to be constant: visions in dull blue and gray; but when certain additives are used, brilliant colours are experienced. Everything appears larger than in real life (macropsia): multitudes of people or animals, often snakes of many colours, and jaguars, dangerous waterfalls or enormous mountains veiled in multicoloured mist or clouds are seen. Very frequently, auditory effects are experienced, especially if chanting or instrumental music is loud. The show of bravado sometimes exhibited at the start of the intoxication does not appear to be common; erotic aspects often reported may be due to the individual personality differences of the participants. Some payés maintain that with the help of the drug they can cause frightening eclipses of the moon, call down tornadoes or control the weather during caapi intoxication.

Muscular incoordination is rarely experienced; in fact, this intoxicant is taken very frequently during dance ceremonies.

The beverage is extremely, sometimes nauseatingly, bitter and vomiting usually accompanies the first draught. It almost always causes diarrhea.

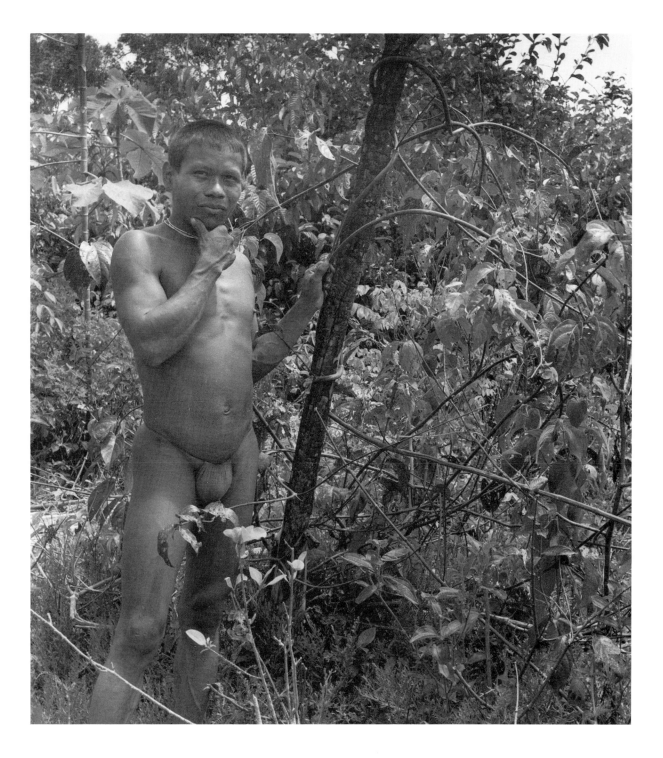

Yajé…stretches back to the beginning of time…

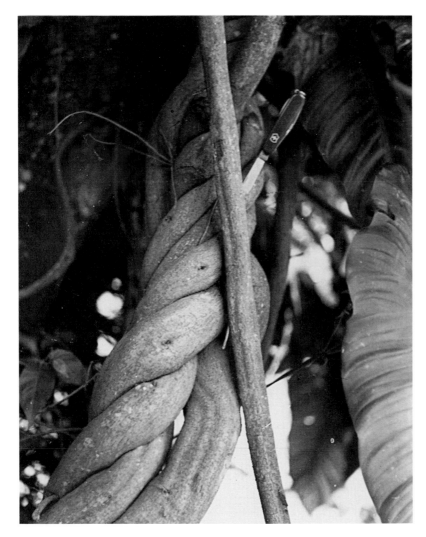

*Banisteriopsis Caapi*, a liana that tends to grow in charming double helices, is one of the primary ingredients in an entheogenic [hallucinogenic] potion known as...ayahuasca, yajé, caapi.... Those who know it call it "spirit vine" or "the ladder to the Milky Way". It is known also as ayahuasca ["vine of the soul"].

H. Rheingold (1989)

...a liana...in charming double helices...

# An eight year old "vine of the soul"

*Cultivated at Fusugasugá, Colombia, from material from the Putumayo*

*Banisteriopsis Caapi* lends itself to cultivation, and many Indians, particularly medicine men, grow the vine near the maloca or in the coca plot. The plant is relatively fast growing, as can be appreciated from the accompanying photograph of an eight year old specimen. The Indians, however, prefer bark from the older and stouter lianas in the forest, maintaining that they are "stronger" in their psychoactive effects.

At the feast of Urubú-coara,
I learnt that caapi was cultivated
...a few hours journey down the
river, and I went there one day
to get specimens of the plants (if
possible) to purchase a sufficient
quantity of the stems to be sent
to England for analysis; in both
objects, I was successful.

R. Spruce (1870)

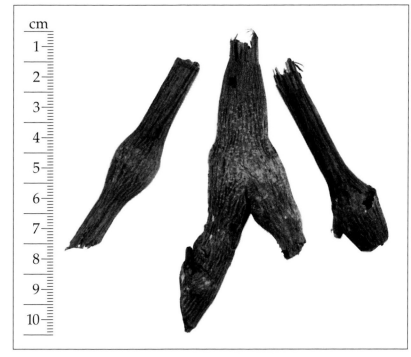

...sent to England for analysis...

## Spruce's original collection of *Banisteriopsis Caapi*

*Río Uaupés, Amazonas, Brazil*

The material collected for chemical analysis by Spruce was de-layed many months arriving in Manáos. Spruce wrote: "thrown aside in a hut [en route down the Río Negro] with only the damp earth for floor...The bundle of caapi would presumably have quite lost its virtue..., and I do not know that it was ever analyzed carefully".

In 1968, it was located in the Royal Botanic Gardens at Kew and finally analyzed 115 years following collection.

The strong physiological action of *Banisteriopsis Caapi* is the result of its content of *beta*-carboline alkaloids, a group of remarkably stable compounds as shown by modern chemical analysis of the specimen collected by Spruce in 1853 which yielded 0.4% of these compounds; this compares favorably with 0.5% found in an authenticated, recently collected specimen.

Often the medicine man will
have a small boy with him,
who may be his son, actual
or adopted, and who is also
credited with magic gifts. Thus
the secrets of the profession
are preserved from generation
to generation...

T. Whiffen (1915)

# Makuna payé and young helper collecting "vine of the soul"

*Oo-ña-mé, Río Popeyacá, Amazonas*

It is not uncommon for medicine men who set out to gather wild vines of yajé to be accompanied by young boys or adolescent males. It is during these forays that they teach the youths the stories concerning the sacred hallucinogen and instruct them in the way to detect the best types. As with other forest plants—*yoco*, for example—these specialists have an uncanny ability to identify numerous "kinds" of the same species, many of which result in being chemically more potent than others but for which botanists can find no morphological characters by which to differentiate these "kinds".

28

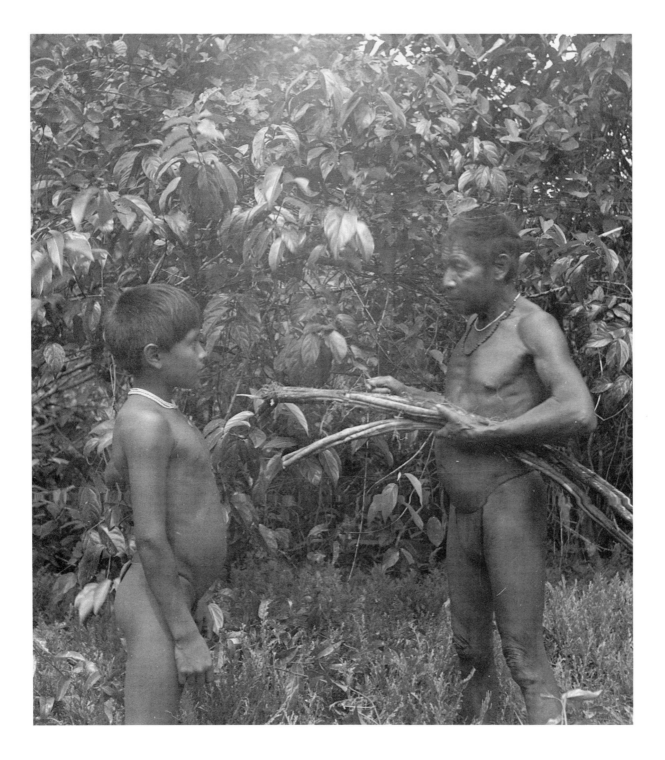

Thus the secrets…are preserved…

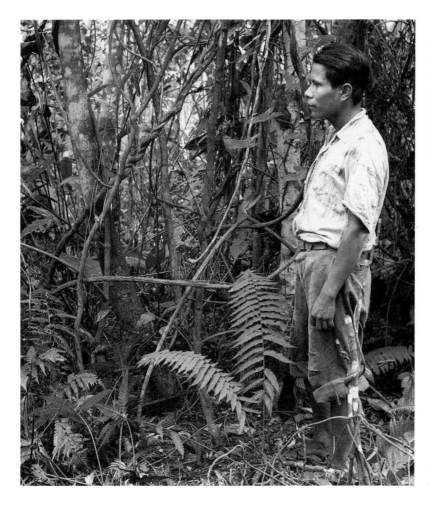

...there is a virtual pharmacopoeia of admixtures [used with ayahuasca]...depending on the magical, ritual or medical purposes for which the drug is being made and consumed.... Many of these admixtures have not been botanically identified, much less characterized.

D.J. McKenna (1986)

...a virtual pharmacopoeia of admixtures...

## Chagropanga is collected usually from the wild

*Mocoa, Putumayo*

One of the most important admixtures to the basic caapi drink, especially in the Colombian and Ecuadorian parts of the Amazon, involves the leaves of another member of the same plant family (Malpighiaceae), *Diplopterys Cabrerana* or chagropanga. The leaves are added to increase the strength and length of the intoxication and are believed to cause the occasional bluish aureole of the visions. This enhancement of effects is the result of the interaction of the tryptamines of *Diplopterys* and the monoamine oxidase inhibiting *beta*-carboline alkaloids of *Banisteriopsis*.

Ayahuasca can be prepared with varying ingredients and of different strengths, from a cold water infusion of the vine alone to a decoction boiled slowly several days in combination with the leaves of the shrub chacruna...

F.D. Lamb (1985)

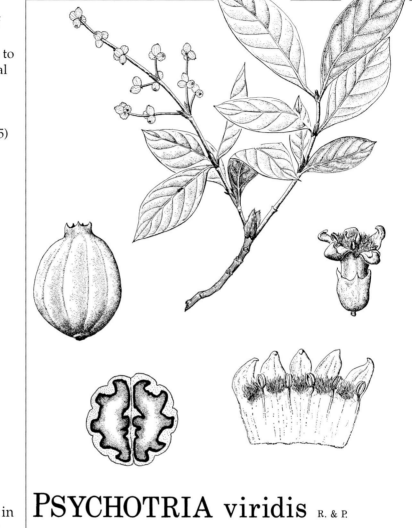

## PSYCHOTRIA viridis R. & P.

Ayahuasca...prepared in combination with...*chacruna*...

# One of the most widely employed additives to ayahuasca

*General in the western Amazon*

*Psychotria viridis* (of the Rubiaceae or Coffee Family), known as chacruna, contains tryptamines which, taken in conjunction with the *beta*-carboline alkaloids present in the "vine of the soul", *Banisteriopsis Caapi*, serve to lengthen and increase the intoxication produced by ingestion of caapi alone.

A...payé explained that the... intense red light of the...resin-covered torch and...from a hearth fire...[is] an important factor in the production of phosphenes and, eventually of true hallucinations.

G. Riechel-Dolmatoff (1975)

## Lighting the torch for the caapi ceremonial dance

*Río Popeyaká, Amazonas*

The eerie effect of the red light and the shadows cast throughout the interior of the great circular maloca combine with the long series of chants offered by the head payé after lighting the torch to begin the feeling of mystery which those who partake of the hallucinogenic drink will experience. Everything seems to cooperate in bringing about the visions, but it is undoubtedly the flickering light and its colour that help to bring on the visions which can be "seen", whether the eyes be open or closed.

Red is perhaps the colour most closely associated with superstition and magic in the northwest Amazonia. There are numerous examples suggesting this association: They include the use of the red saprophytic *Helosis* plant as a styptic; the staining of the payé's hands red with an aroid before his diagnosis of an illness; and the mother's painting red dots on a newborn child's body with achiote, the dye plant *Bixa Orellana*, to make the child strong "like a jaguar".

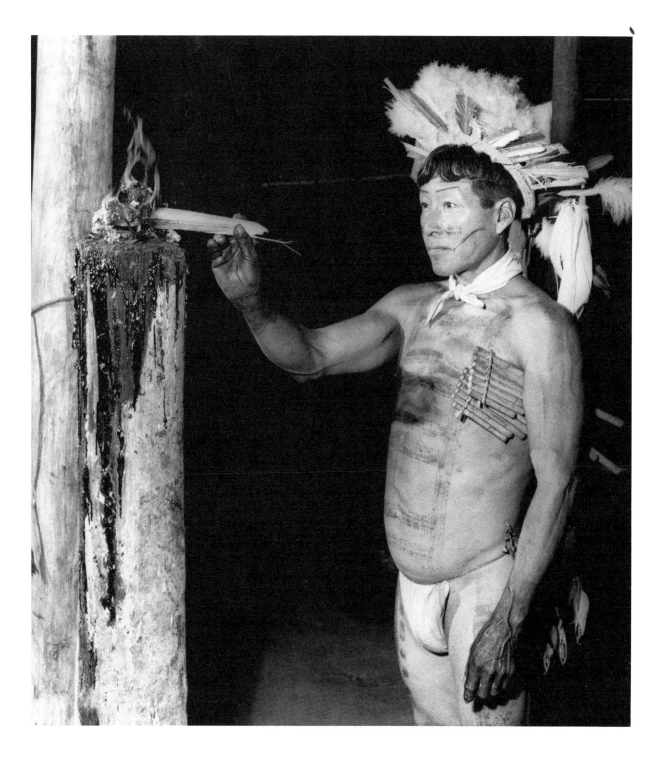

…intense red light…important in the production of…true hallucinations.

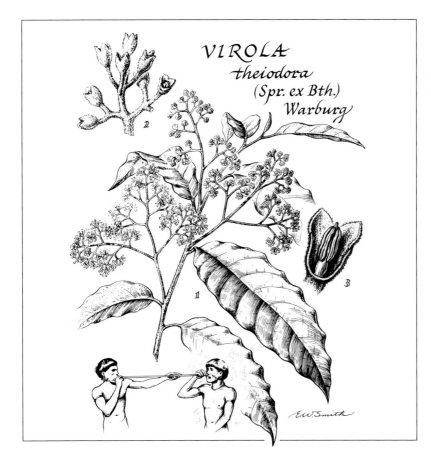

*Viho* (*Virola* snuff) is...an important vehicle of communication with the world of the supernatural. It is employed for medical, magical and prophetic purposes.

F. Trupp (1981)

...communication with... supernatural.

# *Virola* snuff for medicine, magic and prophesy

## *Western Amazonia*

Snuff prepared from the inner bark of several species of *Virola* is extremely important in the life of the Indians of many tribes in the northwest Amazonia of Brazil, Colombia and of the upper Orinoquia of Venezuela. Notwithstanding this importance, it appears for a time to have escaped notice and in the literature was confused with other snuff preparations. It was first mentioned, but without botanical identification, in an anthropological report in 1923 from Venezuela. Definitive identification to species of *Virola* on the basis of specimens collected in Colombia was made in 1954.

The active ingredients in psychoactive *Virola* preparations are tryptamines.

The Myristicaceae is a family of tropical trees.... species of the South American genus *Virola* are an important constituent of the Amazonian forests.

V.H. Heywood, *et al.* (1978)

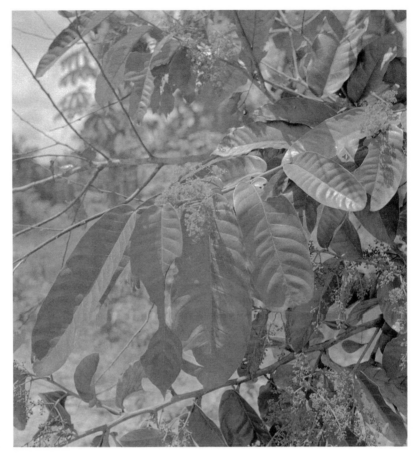

...an important constituent of the Amazonian forests.

## A principal source of *yakee* snuff

*Soratama, Río Apaporis, Vaupés*

The humid tropics of the New World from Central America to the forests of the northern half of South America have some 50 species of *Virola*, a genus of the Nutmeg Family. Four or five species are used as powerful intoxicants by many tribes of South America, either as snuff or as pellets for oral ingestion. The psychoactive principles are tryptamine alkaloids present in high concentration in the exudate of the inner bark. Yakee is the Puinave name for the snuff.

Small amounts of monoamine oxidase inhibitors have been found in *Virola* resin; these enhance the activity of the tryptamines on the central nervous system.

"...the bark is stripped from the trees early in the cool of the morning, and the blood-red resin is scraped from the soft inner bark. The scrapings are kneaded in water, strained and boiled to a thick syrup. When sun-dried, the material is pulverized, sifted and mixed with the ashes of the bark of *Theobroma subincanum* [a wild species of *cacao*].

W.H. Lewis and
M.P.F. Lewis (1977)

## Stripping bark for the resin-like exudate

*Soratama, Río Apaporis, Vaupés*

Several species of *Virola* of the Myristicaceae or Nutmeg Family, particularly *Virola theiodora*, are preferred for preparing hallucinogenic snuff or pellets. Bark is stripped from the lower part of the trunk before the heat of the sun penetrates the forest. A resin-like exudate appears on the inner surface of the bark. This exudate serves other purposes; it is applied to darts as an arrow poison for use in the blowgun; it is also applied over a period of ten to 15 days to areas of skin affected with fungi with an apparent control or cure of the infection.

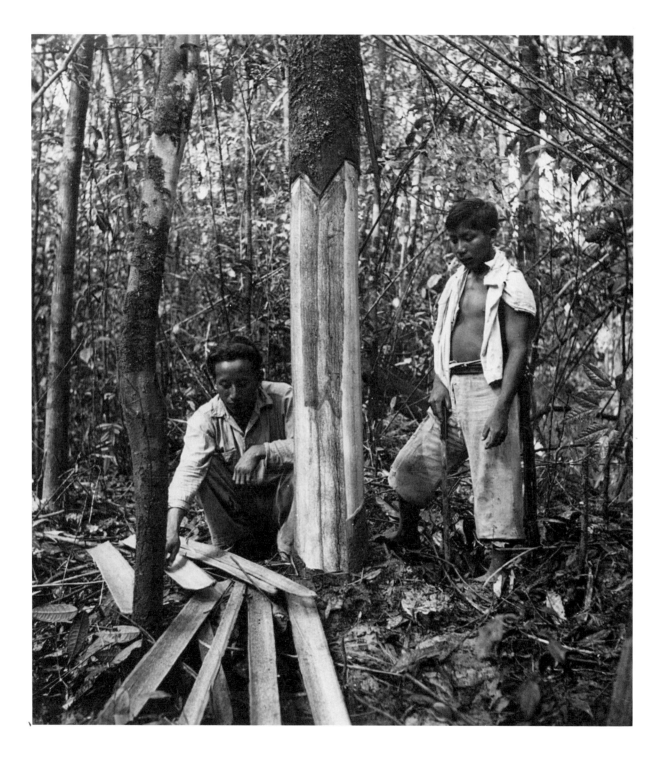

...the bark is stripped...in the cool of the morning...

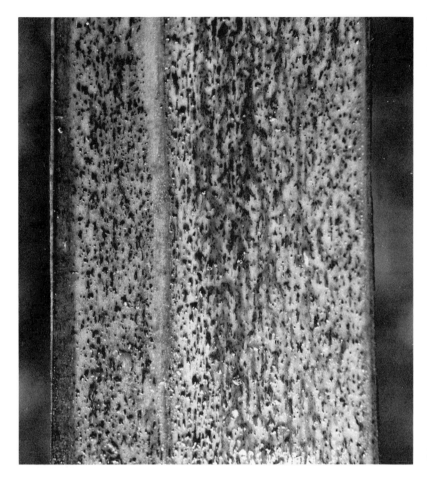

When the bark is stripped, it appears white on its inner side, but only a few seconds later a red brownish resin-like liquid begins to exude in drops. The Indians told us that this "bleeding" is more intensive before the heat of the tropical sun begins to penetrate the forest.

G.J. Seitz (1967)

...a red brownish...liquid begins to exude....

## The copious flow of the exudate is almost immediate

*Soratama, Río Apaporis, Vaupés*

Whether the hallucinogenic preparation from *Virola* constitutes snuff or pellets to be ingested, the first step consists of stripping the bark which results in the appearance of an almost colourless exudate on the inner surface of the bark and the decorticated trunk. This resin-like liquid rapidly turns reddish brown, darkens, and dries to a hard, gummy mass which is scraped off and gathered for further processing.

This exudate contains the tryptamines and other hallucinogenic constituents.

The shaman takes the snuff with the help of a tubular bone... [a] shaman can sniff the powder alone with the help of a fork-shaped snuff machine...various kinds of snuff are kept in separate container[s] made from small shell[s].

F. Trupp (1981)

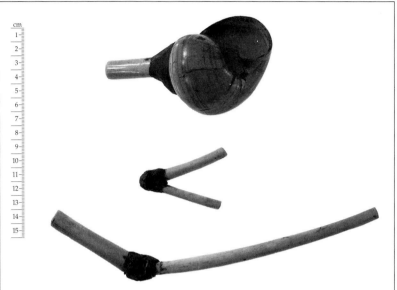

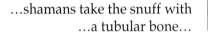
...shamans take the snuff with ...a tubular bone...

## Paraphernalia for making, taking and storing snuff

*Tukanoan and other Indians, northwest Amazonia*

Snuffing is central to the ceremonial practises of the medicine man. Usually, he uses tobacco; but not infrequently, the psycho-active *Virola* snuff is employed.

The application of snuff is often an almost ritual custom, although like tobacco it is also commonly snuffed as a daily habit. Various ingenious methods of snuffing have been developed by the Indians of the northwest Amazon. Both tobacco and the halluci-nogenic snuff prepared from *Virola* employ the same implements which may vary from long tubes (which hold enormous doses) to snuffing tubes prepared from hollow bird bones. Sometimes forked bird bone tubes are used for self administration of the drug. Occasional applications of the powder may be done with the fingers and without implements.

Another snuff, rarely if ever used in the Colombian Amazonia, is prepared from a different psychoactive, tryptamine-containing plant known locally as *yopo*. It is made from the seeds of *Anadenanthera peregrina* of the Leguminosae or Bean Family.

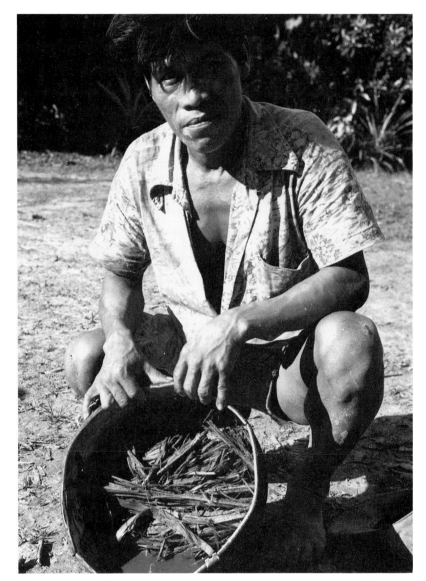

These plants ["magic plants" or hallucinogens]—some of which are medicinal as well as magical—are carefully distinguished from the overwhelming number of purely medicinal plants known to the curanderos [medicine men].

D. Sharon (1972)

...distinguished...from purely medicinal plants...

## Slivers of *Virola* bark ready to boil

*Brillo Nuevo, Río Yaguasyacu, Loreto, Peru*

Amongst those tribes using *Virola* as an oral hallucinogen, the Witotos, Boras and Muinanes, the product may sometimes be employed as a medicine; but, since it is prepared from a very sacred plant, it can be prescribed only by a payé and must be used under his guidance.

...the Witoto, Bora and the Muinane tribes use...*[Virola theiodora]* as an oral hallucinogen, rolling the boiled resin with [an alkaline filtrate of] the ash of *Gustavia Poeppigiana*. Three to six pellets the size of coffee beans induce a hallucinatory experience of several hours in which "little people" are seen, and clarification of problems comes.

W. Emboden (1979)

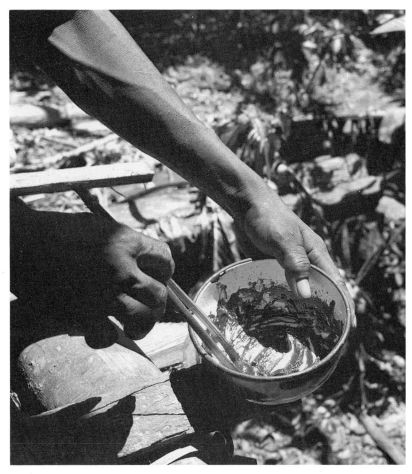

...three to six pellets... induce hallucinatory experience...

## Bora payé whisking boiled *Virola* bark

*Río Yaguasyacu, Loreto, Peru*

The preparation of pellets or pills from the resin-like exudate of the inner bark of *Virola* requires meticulous care in boiling slivers of the bark for at least an hour; constant stirring is necessary. When the resulting paste is thick enough, it is carefully rolled into pellets which are then coated with an alkaline ash and set out to dry. Several different plants may be used to prepare the ash.

Apparently only the Boras, Witotos and Mirañas use *Virola* as an oral hallucinogen. The intoxication induced when half a dozen of these pellets are ingested is not so intense as that caused by *Virola* snuff used by medicine men of other tribes.

41

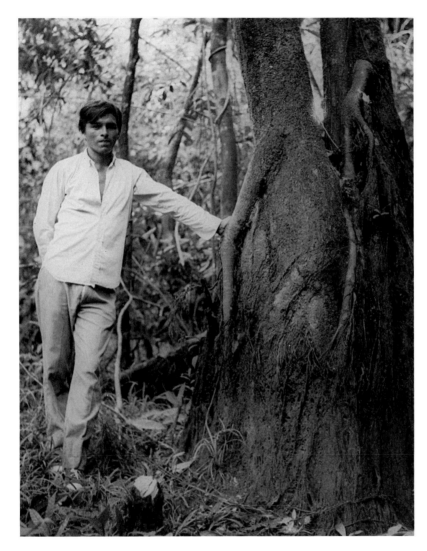

In the family Lecythidaceae, calcium oxalate in the form of single crystals or rosettes is deposited in abundance.

R. Hegnauer 4 (1966)

Calcium oxalate...deposited in abundance.

## An important source of alkaline salt for coating narcotic pellets

*Witotos, Río Karaparaná, Amazonas*

The bark of the tall tree of the Lecythidaceae or Brazil Nut Family, *Eschweilera itayensis*, is favoured for burning to an ash which, when taken up in water, filtered, and the liquid evaporated, yields an alkaline residue used as a "salt" to coat the narcotic pellets prepared from *Virola*. When burned, calcium oxalate in the bark becomes the alkaline calcium oxide.

This plant [*Brunfelsia Chiricaspi*] is considered to be the strongest of a particular class [of *Brunfelsia*] and is preferred for its potent drug effects.... [It]...occurs only in primary forests and is not cultivated...and is known only from the Colombian Putumayo and south to the Río Coca in Ecuador.

T. Plowman (1977)

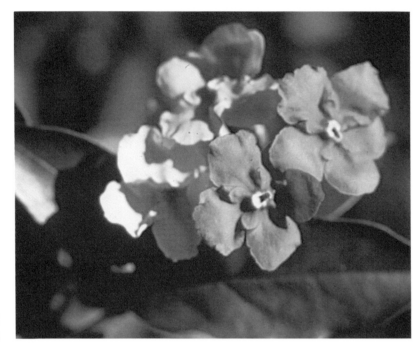

...the strongest... for its potent drug effects

# A powerful but dangerous medicine and hallucinogen

*Puerto Nariño, mouth of Río Loretoyacu, Amazonas*

*Brunfelsia Chiricaspi* is highly valued as a medicine, especially as a febrifuge. Its species epithet comes directly from the vernacular name in the Putumayo—*chiricaspi*—which means "cold tree" or "tree of chills", because it causes a sensation of chills after ingestion. The leaves are often added to the psychoactive drink prepared from *Banisteriopsis*, and it is sometimes employed alone as a hallucinogen amongst the Kofáns, Sionas and Inganos of the Putumayo and adjacent Ecuador

Its use as a hallucinogen, however, seems to be on the wane because of its potent toxicity, causing, in addition to chills and tingling in all parts of the body, dizziness and vertigo, stomach ache, nausea and vomiting, inability to walk and complete lack of muscular coordination. These unpleasant effects withal, Kofán medicine men are reported still to drink a preparation of the leaves, whenever faced with a problem the solution of which they find extremely difficult.

*Brunfelsia* is known to play a part in shamanistic practises.... Shamans often invoke the aid of a particular spirit helper in their healing ceremonies, which may take the form of a bird, snake, insect or plant. Shamans...consider *B. grandiflora* a spiritual guide.

T. Plowman (1977)

# A hallucinogen, medicine, fish poison and spiritual guide

*Region near Mocoa, Putumayo*

This woody shrub is a multipurpose plant found only in the wild. It is employed as an addition to the yajé drink, and in a wide spectrum of therapeutic uses ranging from the treatment of yellow fever to snake bite; like other species, it is valued highly as a febrifuge because of the sensation of chills that follow ingestion. The Siona-Secoyas of Ecuador employ it as an abortifacient.

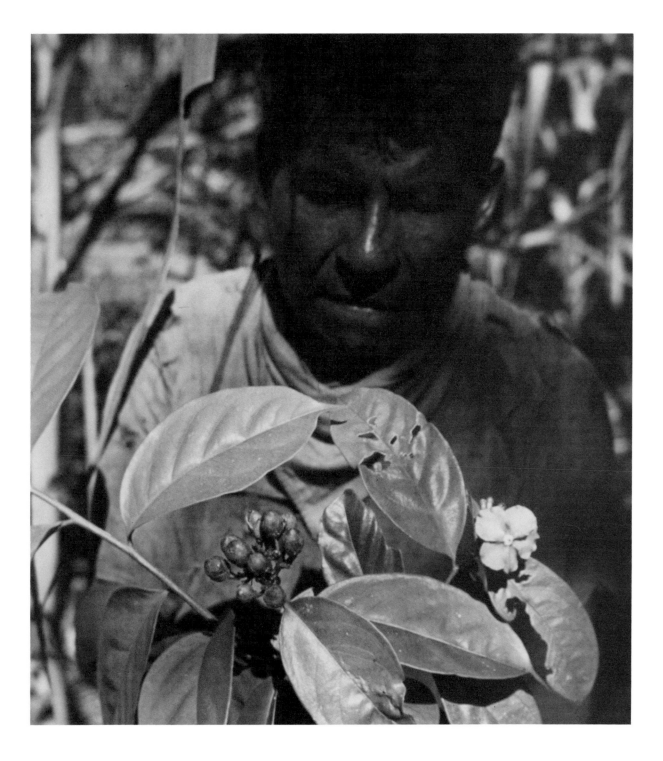

...a spiritual guide.

*Brunfelsia grandiflora* subsp. *Schultesii* is wide-ranging and polymorphic, occurring in western South America from Venezuela south to Bolivia... Since this subspecies is widely cultivated for medicinal and ornamental purposes, some activity of man has undoubtedly influenced its present distribution.

T. Plowman (1973)

# The cultivated form of *chiric-sanango*

*Puerto Nariño, mouth of the Río Loretoyacu, Amazonas*

The principal use of this subspecies is as an additive to the hallucinogenic caapi drink. For this purpose, pieces of the root are preferred, but the leaves may also be employed. It is currently under investigation for possible cardiovascular activity.

This rather scandent shrub is highly toxic to cattle and is a source of concern to owners of cows in the Leticia region, where it is abundant in cultivation or as an escape.

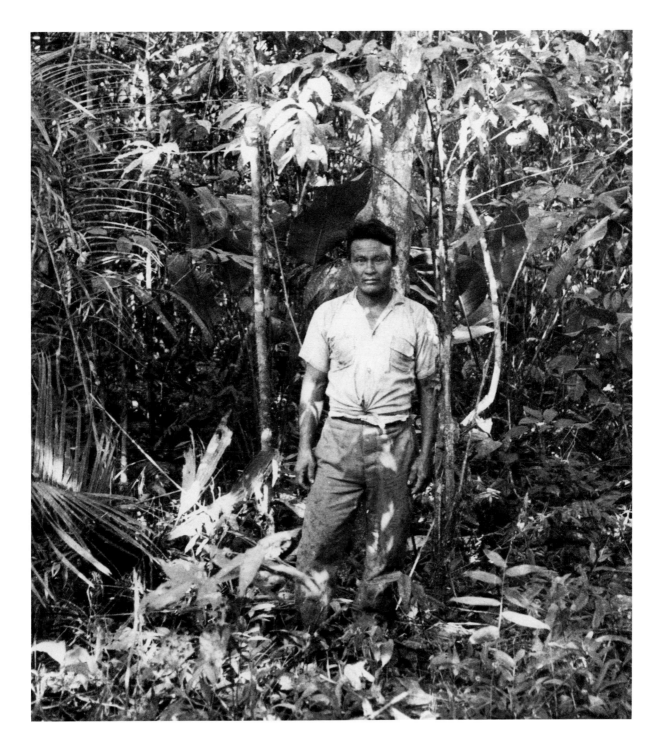

…widely cultivated for medicinal and ornamental purposes…

*Brugmansia* was, and is to a lesser extent today, valued for both its medicinal and psychotropic properties. It was sometimes difficult to separate these two properties in a shamanistic religion where there is...emphasis on malevolent magic and the supernatural cause of illness.

T.E. Lockwood (1979)

# A major hallucinogen in the Andes and western Amazon

*Sibundoy, Putumayo*

*Brugmansia aurea* (formerly known as *Datura candida*) is the major medicinal and narcotic hallucinogen in the Valley of Sibundoy. The "normal" tree is valued; but, as a result of centuries of manipulation by man as a cultigen, it has undergone numerous atrophied forms which are highly esteemed. The normal plant, illustrated, is still highly prized as a medicinal by the Kamsá and Inga medicine men of the Sibundoy Valley.

The most important tropane alkaloids of *Brugmansia* are atropine and scopolamine which antagonise the neurotransmitter acetylcholine, thus depressing bodily functions dependent upon its action. Atropine is used to dilate the pupil in ophthalmology; scopolamine is familiar for its ability to prevent motion sickness. Both may be used in combination to decrease gastric motility and muscle spasm.

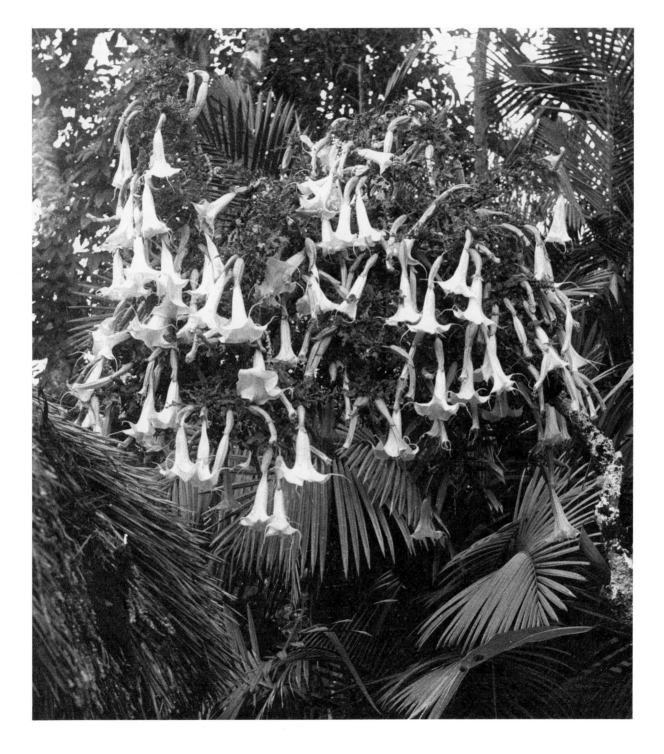

…valued for both its medicinal and psychotropic properties.

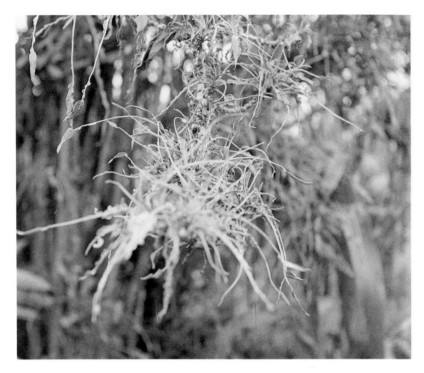

The peculiar characters of the *Brugmansia aurea* cultivars in Sibundoy have resulted from artificial selection of mutations whose induction may possibly be related to virus infection.... [The] rarer cultivars are owned by and known only to the shamans.

T.E. Lockwood (1979)

...cultivars are owned by...the shamans.

## *Kinde borrachero*, a highly atrophied form of *Brugmansia*

*Sibundoy, Putumayo*

There is no satisfactory explanation for the origin in this one locality of the atrophied or aberrant strains of *Brugmansia aurea*. Obviously, the deep interest of the indigenous population in their use in medicine and magic has helped in their preservation. Ten or eleven variants are known by local native names. They may represent incipient "varieties", which would have become extinct had they not appealed so strongly to medicine men. Since the tree is vegetatively propagated, these strains or "varieties" are "owned" by payés, who value them for their bizarre appearance, making them valuable in magic, or for their different physiological effects due, probably, to varying chemical composition.

One of the most highly esteemed of these "clones", with leaves reduced to slender slivers, is known as kinde-borrachero. It is the most widely known and economically important of these cultivars.

The result [of drinking *Brugmansia*] is a narcosis so violent that the participant has to be physically restrained.... Eventually, he will be overtaken by an extended sleep with waking fits of hallucinations and colourful visions that are understood to be communications with the spirit world and souls of the departed. The intent is to become prophetic through divination.

W. Emboden (1979)

...to become prophetic through divination.

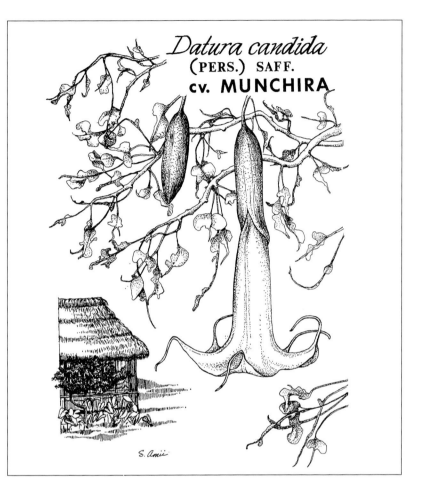

*Datura candida* (PERS.) SAFF. cv. MUNCHIRA

S. Amii

## A curiously atrophied *Brugmansia*

*Santiago, Valle de Sibundoy, Putumayo*

One of the highly prized but rare atrophied clones of *Brugmansia aurea* is *munchiro borrachero*, a stunted plant but which, with age, may attain a height of nine feet. The characteristic of munchira which sets it apart from the other atrophied types of this locality is the shape of the leaves which appear as though irregularly eaten by caterpillars. *Munchira* in the Inga language means caterpillar, referring to the worm-like appearance of the leaves.

According to the local payés, this is one of the strongest of the atrophied Brugmansias, indicative probably of a higher alkaloid content.

...the médicos or curacas take an aqueous maceration of the leaves to produce hallucinations, during which they see the solution of difficult cases of divination, prophesy or diagnosis.

J.F. Theilkuhl (1957)

# An unusually potent hallucinogen of Sibundoy

*Sibundoy, Putumayo*

The Kamsá and Inga medicine men of the Valley of Sibundoy consider this beautiful shrub or small tree, *Methysticodendron Amesianum*, the strongest of all of the solanaceous plants employed as medicines or narcotics in the area. Only the leaves are used in an infusion. The leaves and flowers, when medicinally utilised, are heated in water and plastered on tumours or swellings of the joints. For persistent chills and fever, the whole body is bathed with a warm decoction, followed by rubbing of the chest, back and abdomen with lamb fat.

This is the hallucinogen most preferred by Kamsá payés for divination and prophesy.

*Methysticodendron* is obviously closely akin to *Brugmansia*, and it may not represent a distinct genus but one of the highly atrophied clones of *Brugmansia*, of which there are numerous endemic to the Valley of Sibundoy. Known locally as *culebra borrachera*, it has been considered a cultivar of B. *aurea*. It has also been suggested that its highly atrophied condition is the result of viral infection or the action of a single pleiotropic gene mutation. Not only are the leaves atrophied but the flower is extremely abnormal.

The leaves and stems yield 0.3% of total alkaloids, of which 80% is scopolamine. This relatively high concentration may account for the strong psychotropic activity which the natives attach to this plant.

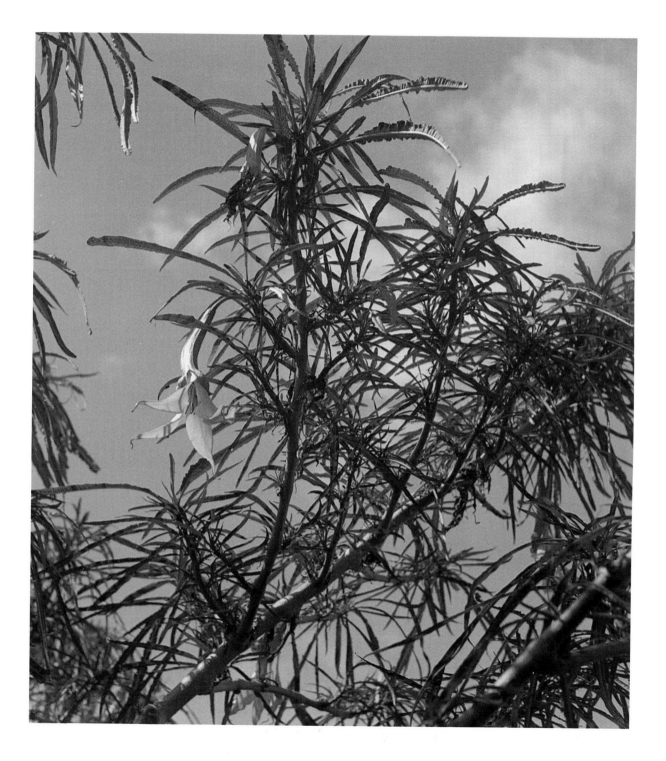

[For]…difficult cases of divination, prophesy or diagnosis.

The sorcerer first leaves the real world and travels to a point above the earth. From "heaven", the sorcerer sees the earth as a huge ball, in contrast to the... belief that the earth is flat. Also, the sorcerer is able to see every person on earth.

J.W. Walton (1970)

## Medicine man after drinking
*munchiro borrachero*

*Santiago, Valle de Sibundoy, Putumayo*

This Ingano payé had, in the previous hour, drunk two cupfuls of a tea prepared from munchira borrachero leaves. The effects were beginning to be evident as he began long and monotonous chanting to his cultivated plant, probably pleading for insight into the cause of a serious illness, apparently advanced tuberculosis, of one of his patients. This dosage would eventually be sufficient to put the medicine man into a trance that might last for four or five hours, during which a young initiate would try to interpret his mumblings, later to inform his teacher.

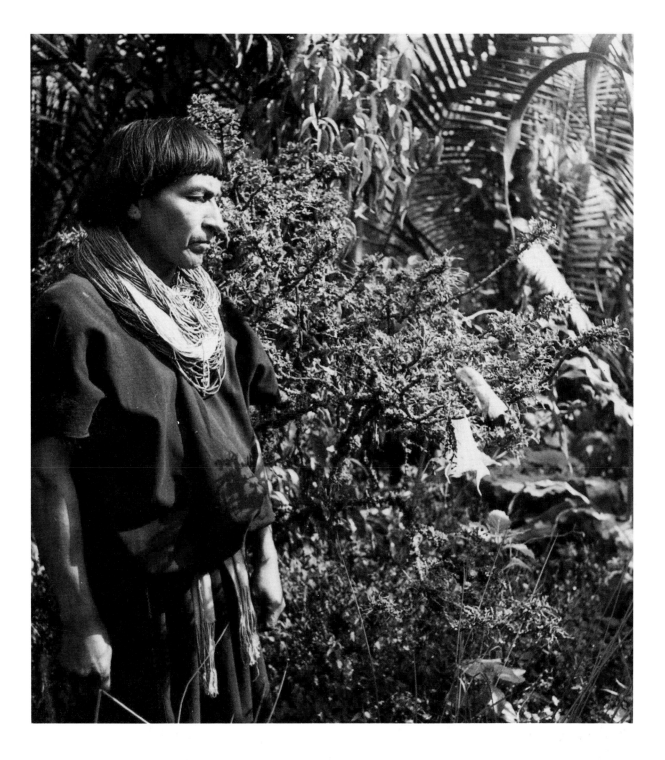

The sorcerer…leaves the real world…

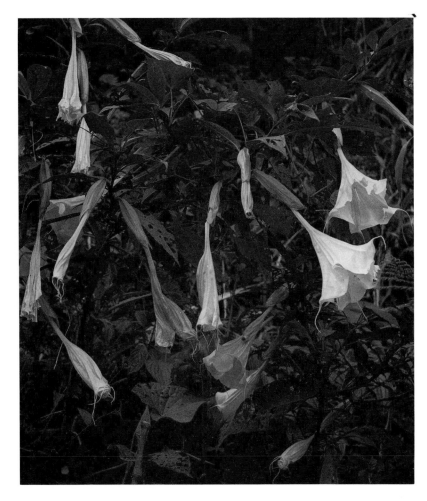

Since the shaman must go into trances with frequency, he does not like to use *Datura*..., because the strength of the plant is such that its repeated use is believed to lead to insanity.

M.J. Harner (1973)

...its repeated use is believed to lead to insanity.

## A principal borrachero (*Brugmansia suaveolens*) from the warm lowlands

*Pepino, Mocoa, Putumayo*

Amongst the Ingano and Siona Indians of the warmer lowlands of the Putumayo, *Brugmansia suaveolens* (formerly known as *Datura suaveolens*) is still used as a medicine and narcotic. It is also added to other drugs of the region, eg., *Banisteriopsis Caapi*.

*Brugmansia suaveolens* is the only species of the genus that grows well in the hot lowlands. Consequently, it is widely employed in the Amazonian regions and along lowland river banks of southern Colombia and Ecuador.

Besides other disagreeable symptoms, these Solanaceae and their active elements, especially atropine and scopolamine, give rise to hallucinations and illusions of sight, hearing and taste.... They are not of an agreeable, but on the contrary, of a terrifying and distressful kind.

L. Lewin (1931)

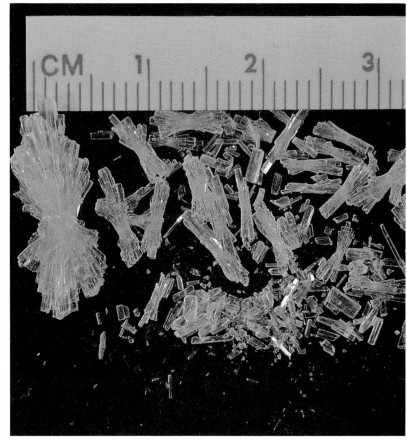

...hallucinations and illusions of sight, hearings and taste...

## Crystals of scopolamine

*Isolated from a Brugmansia species*

The most active hallucinogenic component of the several solanaceous plants used in the western Amazon is scopolamine. It occurs, along with atropine, in various species of *Brugmansia*, *Methysticodendron* and possibly others of the same family.

Plants containing these alkaloids have been used for centuries in other parts of the world as well; the alkaloids themselves have been used in modern medicine for more than a hundred years.

These plants [used by the medicine men] belong to a series of species called "doctores" by local practitioners, because if ingested under certain conditions, they are believed to be able to "teach" the shamans.

T. McKenna (1989)

# Kamsá herbalist-doctor of renown

*Sibundoy, Putumayo*

The medicine men of the Kamsá and Inga tribes of the Valley of Sibundoy have an unusually extensive knowledge of medicinal and toxic plants. They are often seen in the public markets of Bogotá, expounding their knowledge of the treatment of diseases through the use of their plants. One of the most renowned is Salvador Chindoy, who insists that his knowledge of the medicinal value of plants has been taught to him by the plants themselves through the hallucinations he has experienced in his long lifetime as a medicine man. It is such knowledge, fast disappearing, that we must salvage for the potential benefit of all mankind.

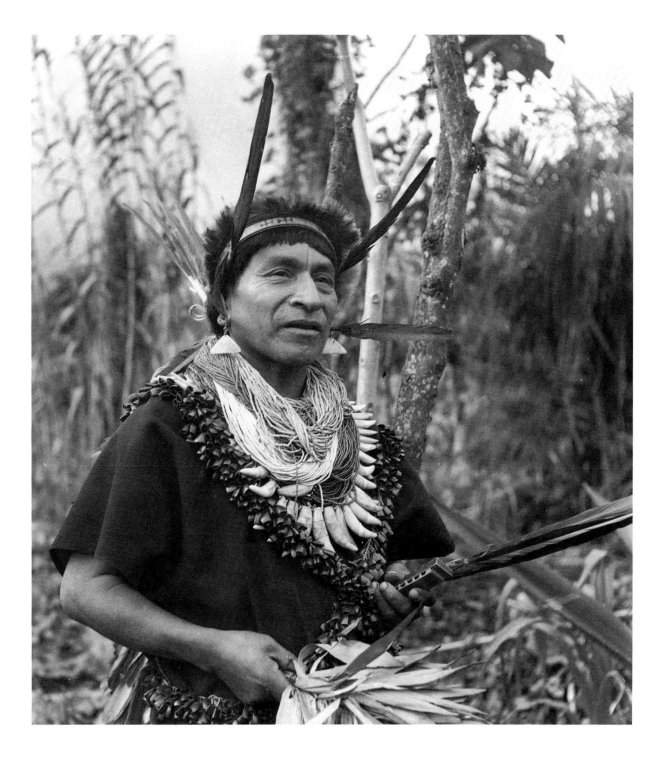

These plants…"teach" the shamans.

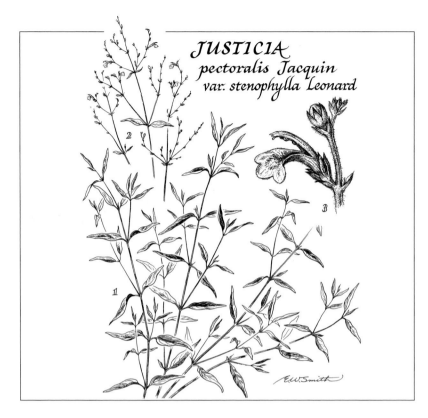

JUSTICIA
pectoralis Jacquin
var. stenophylla Leonard

The whole plant is used in witchcraft, especially in curing practises for serious illnesses... It is cultivated near the houses... the planting and care of it is the responsibility of men, particularly the medicine men.

C. La Rotta (1983)

...used in witchcraft,...

## An aromatic medicinal plant

*Cultivated throughout the northwest Amazonia*

The genus *Justicia* of the Acanthaceae or Acanthus Family, is in need of further scientific investigation. Many or all species are highly aromatic, when the leaves are dried; some are employed medicinally in various parts of the New World tropics.

The Andokes of the Río Caquetá value *Justicia pectoralis* in curative practise for several serious illnesses, and Indians of the Vaupés take a decoction of the whole plant for treating pulmonary problems. *Justicia pectoralis* var. *stenophylla* is widely cultivated in the northwest Amazonia and adjacent Venezuela for use in psychoactive preparations. The dried, aromatic leaves are often mixed with the hallucinogenic snuff made from *Virola*, and it may often be powdered and used alone as a snuff.

Reports of the presence of tryptamines in *Justicia* need corroboration.

The most active physiological compounds isolated and characterized, are withanolides. These chemicals have been shown to possess a wide spectrum of physiological effects...but the use of *Iochroma fuchsioides* as a medicine and hallucinogen in Sibundoy remains unexplained.

M.J. Shemluck (1990)

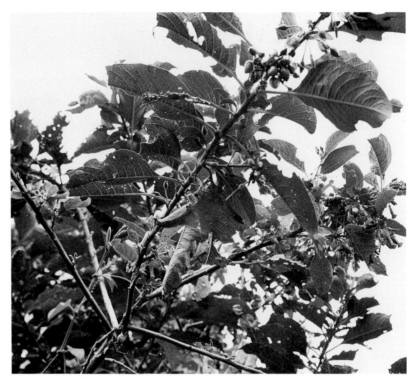

Withanolides...possess a wide spectrum of biological effects...

## A medicine and an intoxicant— *Iochroma fuchsioides*

*Valle de Sibundoy, Putumayo*

The root of this common solanaceous shrub, known locally as borrachero, is reputedly a powerful purgative prescribed by the payés in treating colic, stomach ache, difficulty of digestion or bowel function. The root is rasped and eaten raw with salt when internal injury is suspected following a blow; a tea of the leaves is administered in cases of difficult childbirth.

When the plant is used as a hallucinogen, a tea of the root and leaves is drunk with no admixture. The usual dose is one to three cupfuls over a three-hour period. This psychoactive brew was employed for divination more frequently "in the old days", but according to the medicine men its use is on the wane because of malaise which it causes. A sudorific tea of a bush of the high moors near Sibundoy (*Hedyosmum translucidum*) is taken to relieve this malaise.

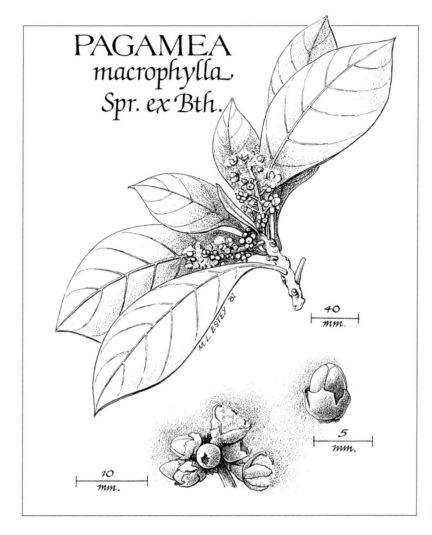

PAGAMEA
*macrophylla*
*Spr. ex Bth.*

M.L ESTEY '81

40
mm.

5
mm.

10
mm.

Thunder owns a special kind of narcotic snuff...which is very potent. It comes in the shape of a hard resin, reddish in colour, and bits of it are scraped off its surface with a piece of quartzite. The resin...must be obtained from thunder and suddenly appears....

G. Reichel-Dolmatoff (1975)

Thunder owns a special…
narcotic snuff…

# A special snuff for divination

*Río Piraparaná, Vaupés*

Barasana medicine men dry and pulverise the resin-rich leaves of the small caatinga tree (of the Rubiaceae or Coffee Family) *Pagamea macrophylla,* and aspirate the resulting snuff during divination ceremonies. This snuff may be the same as the reputedly narcotic snuff which the natives believe is obtained from thunder.

No chemical examination of this species has been carried out. The Makú Indians recognize the plant as toxic but apparently have no use for it.

The leaves are employed as a narcotic and as a stomachic; they are as bitter as gentian; further-more, the Mapuche Indians [of Chile] use them in their textile industries as a yellow dye.

C. Mariani R. (1965)

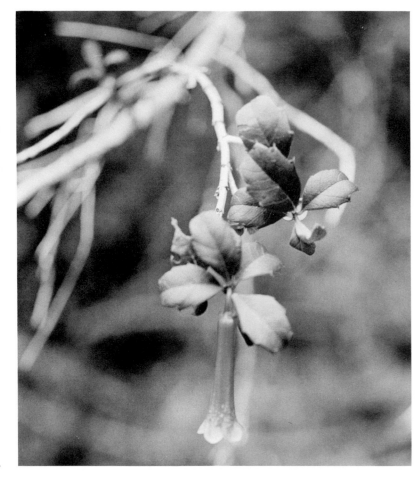

The leaves are…a narcotic…

## An Andean narcotic plant

*Sibundoy, Putumayo*

A recently discovered hallucinogen is *Desfontania spinosa* of the Desfontaniaceae, a small family related to the Loganiaceae, This shrub or low tree occurs from Costa Rica all the way down the Andes to Chile.

Mapuche Indians of Chile employ it as a narcotic; the medicine men of the Valley of Sibundoy in southern Colombia use it when they "want to dream" or "to see visions and diagnose disease". One payé reported that the tea of the leaves is so potent that it makes medicine men "go crazy", for which reason its hallucino-genic use seems to be on the wane in Colombia.

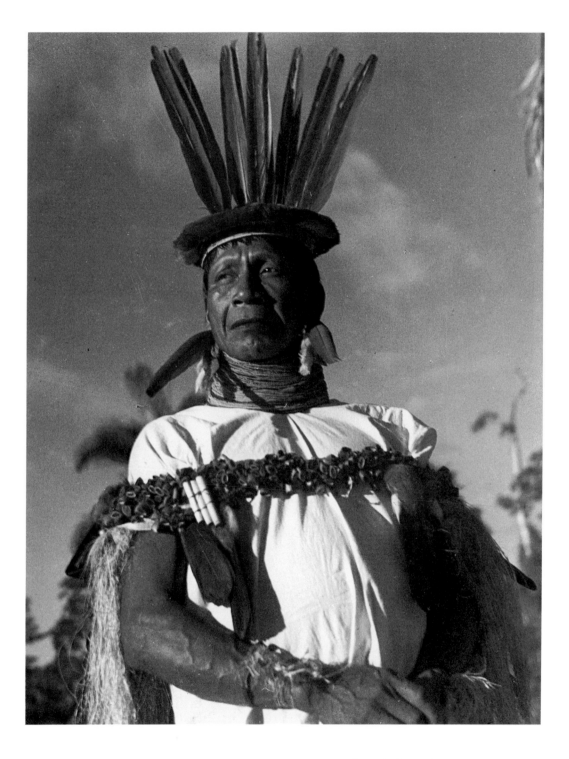

...powers founded on their knowledge of myths.

Shamans are...ranked according to their knowledge and abilities. Their powers are founded upon their knowledge of myths. Most adult men know a considerable number of myths, but shamans differ from the rest, since they know more myths, and...they know and understand the esoteric meaning behind them.... myths are not merely sacred tales or stories but things with inherent power, and it is upon these myths that shamanistic spells are based.

S. Hugh-Jones (1979)

## Kofán medicine man dressed for a ritual

*Porvenir, Río Putumayo, Putumayo*

The Kofáns have more medicine men or payés than any other tribe in the northwest Amazonia. Most of them are deeply knowledgeable men of unusual intelligence and of an imposing personality. The payés are normally expert in manipulating various cosmological forces, and they utilize this ability to solve even socio-political problems and to diagnose and prescribe the cures for most illnesses. They know many plants and they are, almost without exception, "gentlemen of the forest". Some, but not all, claim to be able to travel from one place to another, even at great distances, in an instant and invisibly, but few actually claim to exercise this supernatural ability. Most of them do insist, however, that, when necessary in their trances brought about by hallucinogens, they can change at will into jaguars and later return to the human condition.

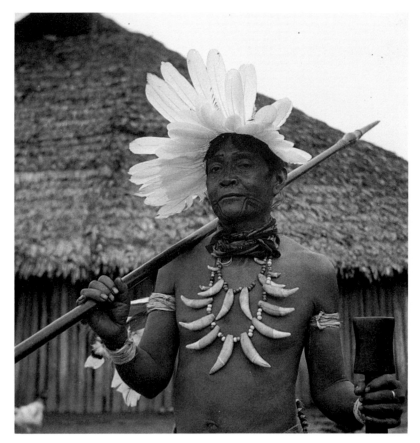

The Sun created various personages to represent him and serve as intermediaries between him and the earth. He charged these intermediaries with protection of Creation and taking care of fertility in life.

G. Reichel-Dolmatoff (1968)

The Sun created various personages to represent him...

# Yukuna payé with his wand of authority

*Caño Guacayá, Río Miritiparaná, Amazonas*

Amongst the Yukunas, the payé is the chieftain. He has a wand of authority and a long rattle which he uses at the beginning of any ceremonial assembly. There are four payés in the Yukuna tribe, all family colleagues. All four believe, as do the medicine men in most tribes of the Colombian Amazonia, that they are charged by the Sun God to care for the well-being of their people.

All shamans are transformers and are said to be able to turn at will into jaguars, huge serpents, harpy eagles or other fearful creatures.... Jaguar transformation is achieved through the absorption of a powerful narcotic snuff [*Virola*].... Prostrate in the hammock he will growl and pant, strike the air with claw-like fingers, and those present will be convinced that his wandering soul has turned into a blood thirsty feline.

Reichel-Dolmatoff (1968)

...his wandering soul has turned into a blood thirsty feline.

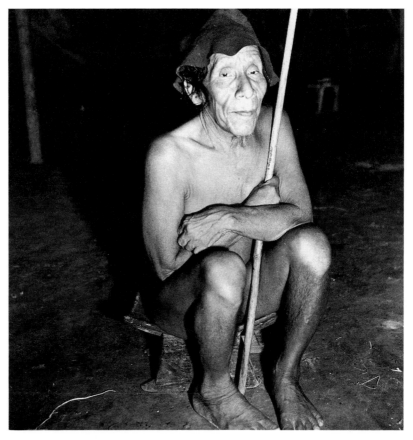

# Famous Yukuna medicine man

*Caño Guacayá, Río Miritiparaná, Amazonas*

The position of payé is usually not hereditary, although many times a son of a medicine man may follow in his father's footsteps. Much more important in the tribes of the northwest Amazonia are an individual's psychological and educational characteristics, some or most of which he could learn through youthful apprenticeship to a payé. He must be willing to undergo constant dedication to his service to the tribe; he must have an excellent memory for the many chants and songs he must know to initiate ceremonies; he must be willing to pass nights without sleep, to fast often and to be willing occasionally to practice sexual abstinence. Most important of all, for most payés, he must be willing to take hallucinogens and to "understand" the visions which they bring about.

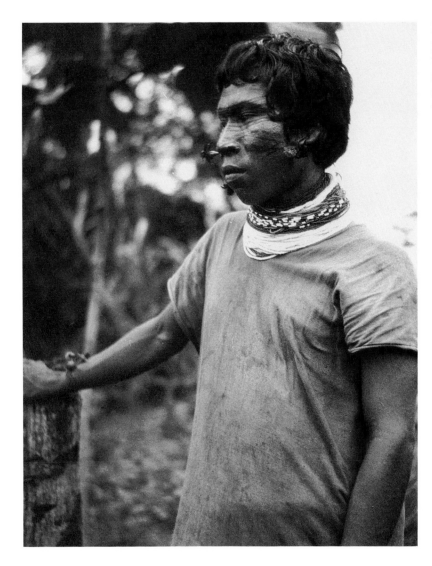

Items of adornment, such as face painting, tattooing and ear plugs were badges of tribal membership, sex, society affiliation or class status, according to tribal patterns they entered.

J.H. Steward (1949)

...badges of...class status...

## Siona medicine man with facial tattooing

*Ucursique, Putumayo*

The accoutrement of payés differs from tribe to tribe or from one individual to another. In many cases, a medicine man may not wear any special badge of his status. Amongst the Sionas, one of the principal shamans indicates his position through facial tattooing. In the Vaupés, certain intricate feather crowns are worn in dances or other shamanistic ceremonies, although feather work is worn often by male participants who are not payés.

Religion and medicine centre in the cult of payé men, who supposedly have the power to call down lightning, change the weather, transform themselves into jaguars, shoot magic stones that kill or sicken and cure disease.

P.H. Allen (1947)

Religion and medicine centre in the cult of payé men…

## A Yukuna payé in full regalia

*Caño Guacayá, Río Miritiparaná, Amazonas*

Amongst the Yukunas and Tanimukas of the Río Miritiparaná, payés still wield a mighty influence. The Yukunas, once a powerful group, and the terror of the neighboring tribes, are now a small but compact unit which numbers probably fewer than 300. The tribe is divided into two groups: the People of the Boars, the most warlike in the old days but now numbering 30 or 40 individuals; and the People of the Eagles. Both now live amicably together, speak the same language and have payés equally respected.

A powerful payé of the Eagles acts usually as chief of the Kai-ya-ree and of other sacred ceremonies such as the We-ra, a dance performed without uniforms—the men in their traditional *guayuco* ("breech cloth"), but with very ornate and beautiful head-dresses. In this dance, celebrated for the Spirit of the Waters, the payé or chieftain goes up and down the rivers blowing loud blasts on a trumpet and later beats messages on the *manguaré*.

69

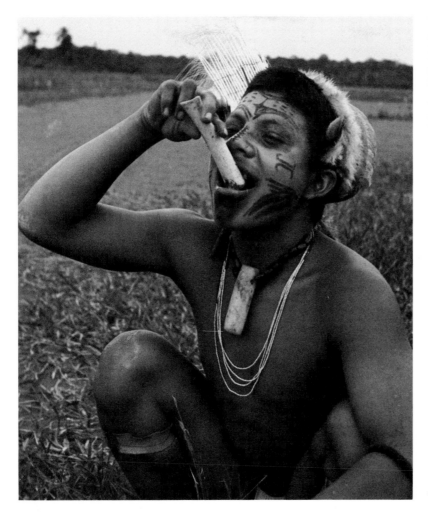

Widespread shamanistic possessions...include gourd rattles, carved wooden stools, plant emetics and crystal rocks, which latter are constantly worn or carried about for use in curing practices.

R.H. Lowie (1949)

...crystal rocks...constantly worn...for curing...

## Makuna payé, with badge of status, taking coca

*Río Piraparaná, Vaupés*

Special decorations, often used by payés amongst the Tukanoan tribes of the Vaupés, are white quartz crystals worn hanging around the neck. These crystals are eagerly sought in the rapids of the uppermost Río Orinoco and the Río Taraira.

These rocks are valuable possessions and are passed down from one generation to the next; they have very powerful supernatural influences, according to the payés.

They have also wisemen or wizards among them, of great esteem; who serve them as counsellors as well as for Religion and Physick as for Law and Policy; and in the year 1639, (they) found an Indian in these Countries that called himself the son of the Sun, who...said that every night he went...to consult the Sun for the government of the following day.

Count of Pagan (1663)

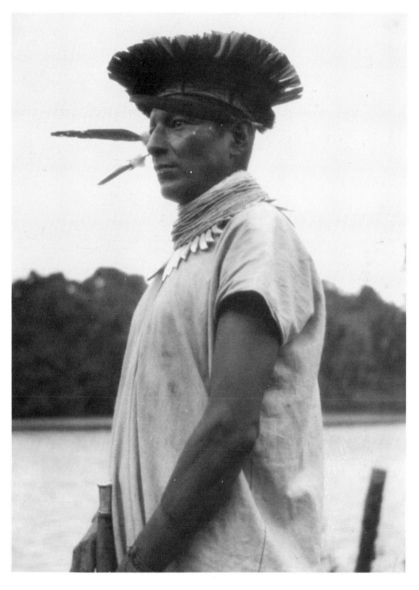

...[he} called himself the son of the Sun...

## Principal payé of the Kofáns

*Río Sucumbios, Putumayo*

This Kofán is both the payé and chieftain of the group living on the creek called Conejo. He is highly respected by all Kofán groups in the Putumayo and adjacent Ecuador and by Colombian settlers in the region. He has rightly been called "a gentleman of the forest".

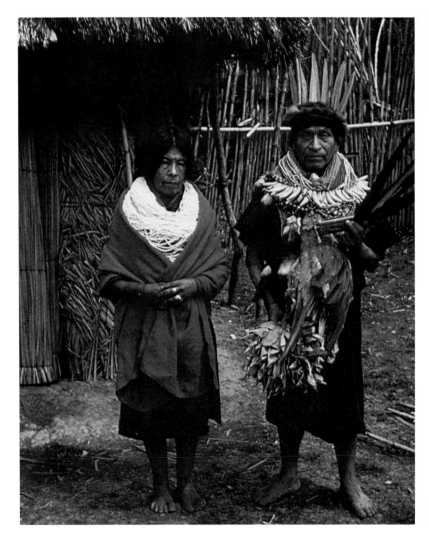

Medical treatment is in the hands of selected men, sometimes also old women, who are distinguished by their powers of observation, cunning and management of their occupation.

T. Koch-Grünberg (1909)

...sometimes...women... distinguished by powers of observation...

## Kamsá medicine man and his wife

*Sibundoy, Putumayo*

It is often the women who know most about wild medicinal plants and who often collect them for the payé or for general use by members of the maloca. Not infrequently, male members of the tribe who have suffered a minor wound will consult a woman herbalist instead of a payé. Occasionally, the herbalist may be the wife of the shaman. Knowledge of plants with bioactive activity when ingested is usually rather widespread in the non-shamanistic circles of most of the tribes.

The medicine man, holding a calabash rattle in his left hand, shakes it continually over the prostrate patient. Then he takes occasional puffs at a large cigar, which he holds in his right hand, and blows the tobacco smoke over the patient's body.... Slowly and rhythmically, he strokes the patient, so that he can draw the "disease matter" out of his body. Having seized this disease matter, he throws it into the air and then disperses it by blowing tobacco smoke in all directions; throughout his ministrations, the medicine man intones a slow, monotonous chant.

P. Radin (1942)

Slowly and rhythmically, he...can draw {out} the "disease matter"...

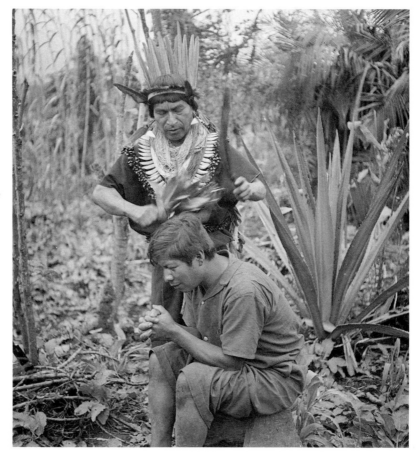

## Famous Kamsá payé at work

*Sibundoy, Putumayo*

Perhaps the most renowned payé in the western Amazon of Colombia is Pedro Chindoy, a member of the Kamsá tribe. Not only is his fame known far from his village in adjacent parts of the Amazonia of Colombia and Ecuador, but he travels every year, practicing his art and selling medicinal herbs; he is very frequently seen in Bogotá and Quito.

Pedro Chindoy has for many years been friendly to and cooperative with botanists and anthropologists who visit Sibundoy. Those of us who have had contact with him are convinced that he really believes that his techniques produce results, and we cannot find a shred of duplicity in his dealings.

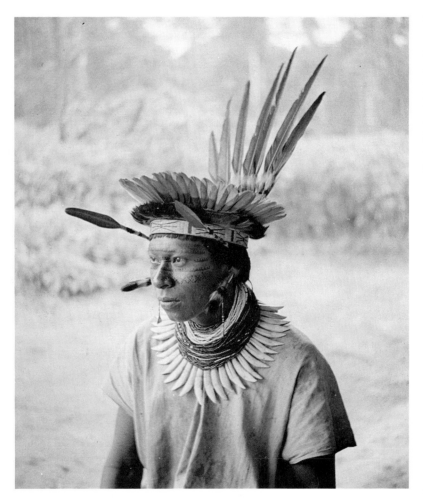

They ascribe a direct intercourse with the demons to their payé, who is acquainted with many powerful herbs...in extraordinary cases, he is applied to for his advice, which he gives after consulting the demons.... The payé administers many medicines which are often prepared with magical ceremonies.

J.B. von Spix and
C.F.P. von Martius (1824)

...acquainted with many powerful herbs...

## Kofán herbalist and payé

*Río Sucumbíos, Putumayo*

Knowledge of the properties of plants is particularly characteristic of Kofán payés. Occupying the westernmost part of the Amazon at the foot of the Andes in the Colombian Putumayo and adjacent Ecuador, this tribe lives in an extremely species-rich flora. They use more kinds of plants, for example, in preparing arrow poisons than any other tribe in the Colombian Amazonia. Although their superstitious beliefs are extremely complex and effective in the practice of their art, their knowledge of how to prescribe plant drugs is extraordinary, and they employ plants more than payés in most tribes of the region.

The shaman is an old man or woman who has established communion with the soul of a deceased person, an animal spirit or a supernatural monster.

B.J. Meggers (1971)

The shaman is an old man
or a woman…

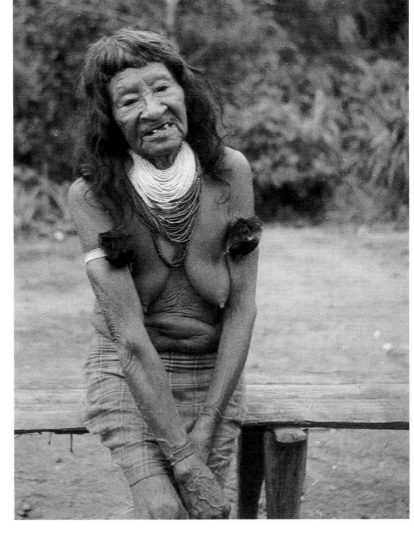

## An elderly Tikuna medicine woman

*Río Amacayacu, Amazonas*

In some tribes, a woman may acquire extensive knowledge of plants; and occasionally she capitalises on this knowledge, becoming fearsome, particularly amongst the young who believe that she is able to hex people through the power of her powdered tobacco and toxic plants which, accompanied by magical incantations, she blows over a patient's body. Some of these female payés do actually prescribe plants which have alleviatory properties.

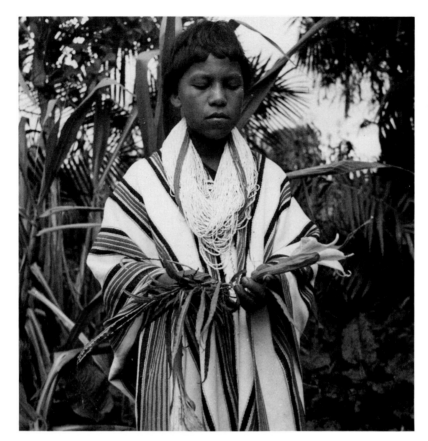

...the people who know the most about traditional botanical medicine—the shamans—claim that their knowledge is derived directly from the plants as well as from their human teachers.

H. Rheingold (1989)

...knowledge...directly from the plants...

## Kamsá beginner in shamanistic knowledge holding favourite hallucinogen

*Sibundoy, Putumayo*

The principal payé of the Kamsá Indians of Sibundoy has often cooperated with numerous western botanists, Colombian and foreign, who have worked in this highland, mountain-girt valley, near where one of the major Colombian Amazonian tributaries originates. He insists that his knowledge and power come to him directly from the plants themselves through hallucinations. His student is photographed holding one of the most bioactive hallucinogens of this mountain valley, where high endemism prevails and where more psychoactive plants are known and used than probably in any other locality in South America, if not in the world. This young Kamsá native reflects the seriousness of those who prepare for study with the principal payé of Sibundoy.

76

The office of payé is not hereditary ...More important than family tradition...are certain psychological and intellectual qualities... recognized in his youth. Among these qualities are a deep interest in myth and tribal tradition, a good memory for reciting long sequences of names and events, a good singing voice and the capacity for enduring hours of incantations during sleepless nights preceded by fasting and sexual abstinence. Above all, a payé's soul should "illuminate;" it should shine with a strong inner light rendering visible all that is...hidden from ordinary knowledge and reasoning. This supernatural luminescence... is said to manifest itself when he ...sings or...explains...hallucinatory experiences.

G. Reichel-Dolmatoff (1975)

...certain...qualities... recognized in his youth.

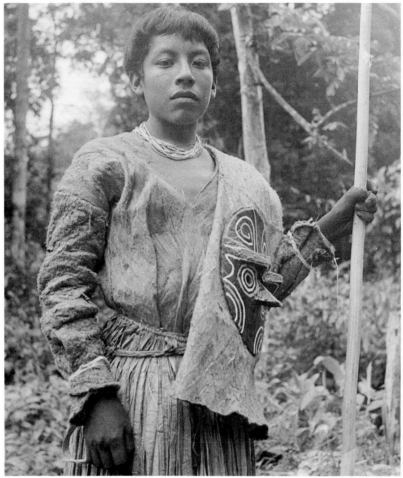

# Tanimuka student preparing for shamanism

*Río Miritiparaná, Amazonas*

Any youth showing extraordinary interest in animals or hunting—such as this Tanimuka boy—may apply to become a payé's student or helper. Knowledge of the habits and lairs of animals is more or less general knowledge amongst male members of these tribes, but when this knowledge is combined with interest in the mythological or superstitious beliefs concerning animals, particularly those associated with jaguars and anacondas, practicing payés may try to interest a youth in becoming a student, even when he may be deficient in some of the other necessary qualifications.

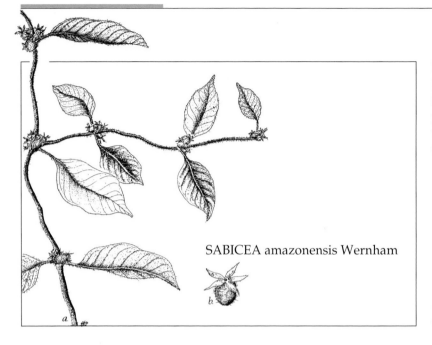

SABICEA amazonensis Wernham

Before the tipping out of the fruit [in the initiation ceremony], the initiates were each given small pink berries of the *kana* vine... which had previously been blown over by the shaman.

S. Hugh-Jones (1979)

...pink berries...blown over by the shaman.

# A ritualistically important vine

*Common throughout the Colombian Amazonia*

Kana, *Sabicea amazonensis* (Rubiaceae), is one of the payé's most important plants, despite its unpretentiousness. It grows almost as a weed around human habitations.

The reddish berries are sometimes added to the normally bitter caapi drink to sweeten it. Youthful initiates into manhood are given kana fruits to eat when they take their first drink of caapi which has been made especially strong.

Payés maintain that "each fruit is a heart, and the vine with the fruit is...a series of hearts on a string. The hearts are those of each generation connected together by an umbilical cord, the vine. This cord is said to extend out from the house and...down the river to the east...where the sun comes from, the source of all humanity. By eating this fruit, the initiates become connected to the ancestral source of life by an umbilical cord, the river".

The payé blows over the red berries and offers them to a new born baby, and the fruit is involved in magical treatment concerning the mother's milk.

Nothing is known of the chemistry of *Sabicea*.

The novitiate [for payé status] lasts from one month to five.... The novitiate consists of four sections: abstinence, insertion of magical substances into the body, learning of songs and ritual and examinations. The abstinences include sexual relations and the eating of fish, broiled game flesh and...pineapple...the novice, who is expected to become thin, lives on nothing but manioc and water.

I. Goldman (1963)

The novice...lives on... manioc and water.

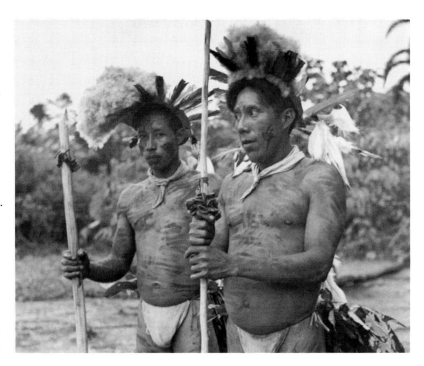

# Tukano aspirants for medicine man status

*Río Papurí, Vaupés*

Boys take preparation to become payés seriously and, since there may be several in a given region or tribe who are in training, there is often fraternal comradeship amongst them. The "courses" vary from payé to payé and not infrequently may last for two years or even longer. In addition to deprivation of usual foods, play and sexual activity, the basic content of the training includes very frequent use of hallucinogens, usually the "vine of the soul", and discussions with the payé-teacher of the visions and other experiences. The boys must also learn endless incantations concerning the mythological history of the tribe and the various spirits and supernatural masters with whom the initiate must know how to converse. Study includes the superstitions associated with plants, animals, waterfalls and rapids, petroglyphs and many other aspects of the payés stock-in-trade. Some payés, especially those who undertake actual treatment of illnesses, instill in their students an extensive understanding of medicinal plants, their recognition and the proper period of the year or hour of the day for their collection and dosage.

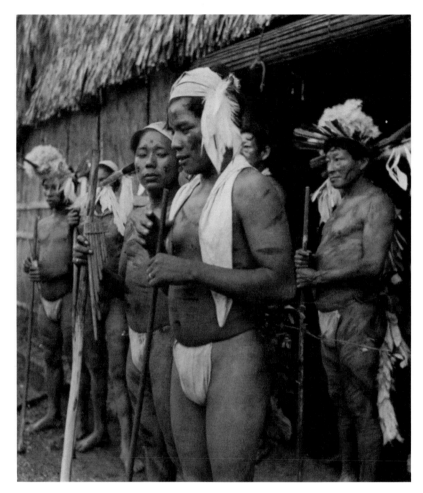

Initiation into the priesthood was not easy and required considerable fortitude.... The first thing the instructor prepared was some tobacco juice, and each candidate was then given a large calabash of tobacco water to drink and a cigarette to smoke. Before the effects were apparent, they were taught how to make the rattle.

P. Radin (1942)

Initiation...required considerable fortitude...

## Kubeo dance of initiation into shamanistic status

*Río Kubiyú, Vaupés*

When training for the status of payé has been concluded, there is a "graduation ceremony" or dance. The payé-teacher, proud of his students, officiates at the affair in full regalia, usually giving the young men feathered crowns, beads, rattles or other insignia that they can use in the practice of their art. The dances, often lasting two or three days, are attended by the entire population residing within a reasonable distance. At these ceremonies, it is usual for all adult males to partake of the "vine of the soul", snuff tobacco and drink chicha.

...the process of education and learning, especially in matters related to religion and ritual, continues throughout their lives.

S. Hugh-Jones (1979)

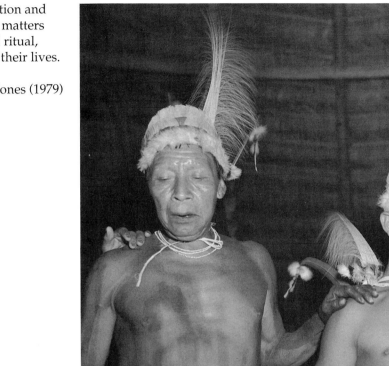

...education and learning ... continues throughout their lives.

# Makuna payé with his former student

*Río Piraparaná, Vaupés*

This medicine man, of great fame in the region for his "cures", often travels long distances when his services are requested. In this photograph, he is dancing and chanting with one of his former students who recently became a payé. They are both under the influence of the "vine of the soul" and are trying to diagnose the cause of the illness of a youth lying on the ground with epilepsy-like symptoms.

A greater keenness becomes apparent in all the senses... smell, sight, hearing and touch all participate.... It is then that the hallucinations begin. One by one, external objects assume strange appearances...sounds are clad in color, and colors contain a certain music.

C. Baudelaire (1971)

# Kubeo medicine man under caapi intoxication

*Mitú, Río Vaupés, Vaupés*

Of all the hallucinogenic plants employed around the world in aboriginal ceremonies and religions, there is perhaps none that causes so many bizarre psychic effects as *Banisteriopsis*, "the vine of the soul". There can be no wonder why any plant with such unworldly powers has been accepted as sacred. One of the unique characteristics of caapi intoxication is its lack of interference with muscular coordination, even at the height of its excessive imbibition, unless, of course, a considerable amount of alcoholic chicha be taken during the dance. Caapi is usually prepared alone, without plant admixtures; sometimes, other plants with different chemical constituents are added to the drink. In both cases, the lack of interference with muscular activity is striking.

Another uniqueness of caapi intoxication is the ability of the participant to experience the effects, particularly the visionary effects, in the light of day or in the lighted malocas.

The kinds of visual hallucinations and their intensity vary and, as with other aboriginally employed hallucinogens, are undoubtedly conditioned by social or superstitious beliefs. That jaguars and anacondas are very frequently "seen" may be due to the widespread acceptance of the belief that the shaman can turn into a jaguar at will and that the anaconda figures prominently in the superstitions and religion of the western Amazonia. These two animals have acquired their roles in mythology and superstition because they are the two most feared animals of the forests, due to their stealth and power.

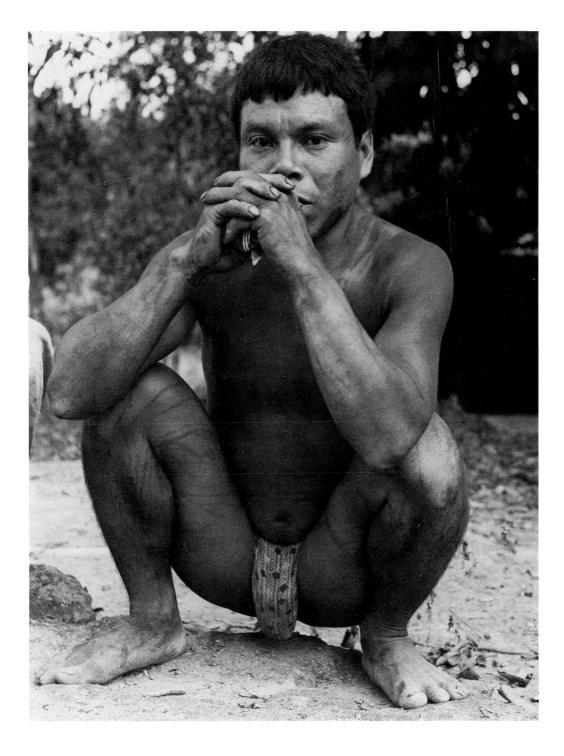

...the hallucinations begin.

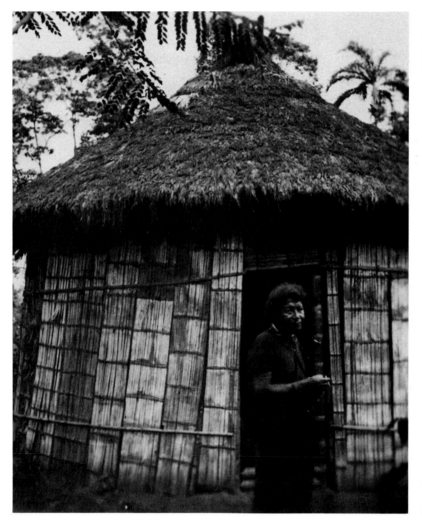

These...payés don't live in the malocas with the rest of the tribe but in little huts apart in the jungle.

G. MacCreagh (1926)

These payés...live...
apart in the jungle.

# Ingano medicine man and his private "office"

*Mocoa, Putumayo*

In many tribes, some payés live with their families in the maloca; but others, especially the elderly ones, may sleep in a hut removed from the site of the principal house. Many of their consultations with patients and private rituals will take place in such a tiny hut. All major ceremonial practices, however, will take place in the maloca, usually during specific dances, or even in the open space surrounding it.

One of the most typical aspects of the shamanistic experience is the change into another state of consciousness, often called a trance, with the shaman feeling that he is taking a journey.

M.J. Harner (1973)

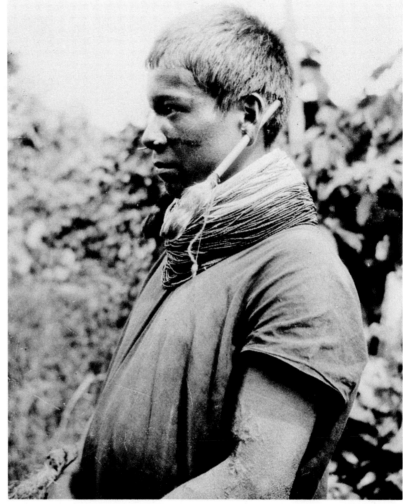

...the shaman...
taking a journey.

## Kofán payé under influence of the "vine of the soul"

*Conejo, Río Sucumbios, Putumayo*

The effects of the "vine of the soul" may be experienced at the beginning of the sacred intoxication but also can be prolonged, especially if other psychoactive additives be combined with the drink. The effects often begin almost immediately, even if the drug be taken during daylight.

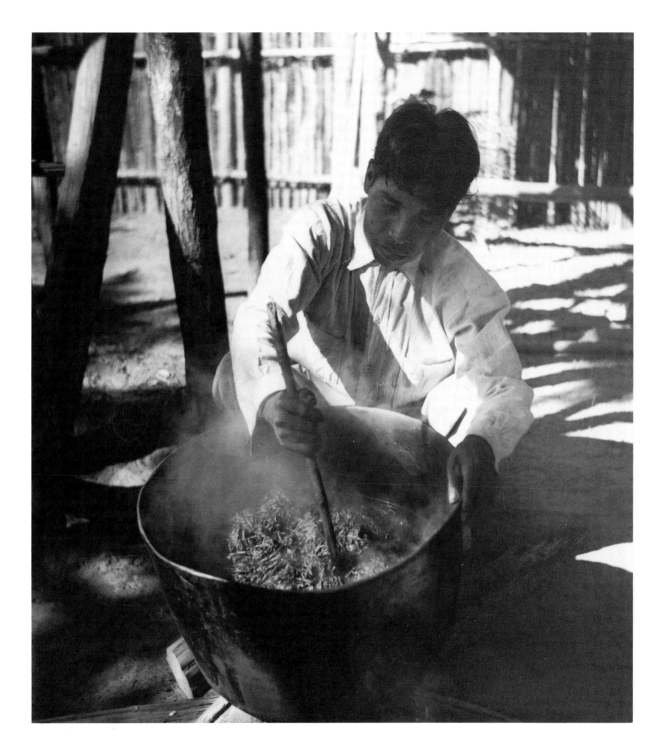

...leaves are boiled...to a concentrated liquid...

...tobacco leaves are boiled down to a concentrated liquid...it acquires the consistency of thick molasses—that is *ambíl*.... Tobacco enters very much into...[the] shamanistic and general magico-religious complex.

J. Wilbert (1987)

## Witoto boiling tobacco to prepare *ambíl*

*La Chorrera, Río Igaraparaná, Amazonas*

There are few plants more important in South American shamanism, whether as medicines or in mythology, than tobacco: *Nicotiana Tabacum* of the Solanaceae or Nightshade Family. It is native to the Andes. South American Indians had long ago discovered every way of utilizing it: smoked, as a snuff, chewed, licked, as a syrup applied to the gums, and in the form of an enema. In many tribes, payés use tobacco smoke blown over a sick patient, especially on the area theoretically affected, with appropriate incantations in the belief that this practice can cure of itself or at least serve as a prelude to other treatments.

One of the marvielles of this Hearbe...is the maner how the primitives of the Indias did use of it...when there was amongst the Indians any maner of business... thei wente and propounded their matter to their chief Prieste; Forthewith...he toke certain leaves of the Tabaco and caste them into the fire and did receive the smoke ...at his mouthe and at his nose with a Cane; and in takying of it he fell doune uppon the grounde as a dedde manne...and when the hearbe had doen his woorke he did revive and awake and gave theim their answeres according to the visions and illusions which he sawe.... In like sorte the reste of the Indians for their pastyme doe take the smoke...for to make themselves drunke withall....

N. Monardes (1572)

# Yukuna students of shamanism taking tobacco snuff

*Caño Guacayá, Río Miritiparaná, Amazonas*

Tobacco is essential in the training of young men wishing to be payés. This aspect of their training is present in virtually every tribe in the Colombian Amazonia.

Amongst the Yukunas, for example, students must snuff tobacco in large amounts. It may take several years of this training before they master the knowledge of the payé and before they satisfy him of their proficiency.

The tobacco plant and the methods of its use amongst New World Indians never ceased to astonish the earliest European "explorers". It was unknown, of course, in the Old World before 1492, and snuffing was unknown in the Eastern Hemisphere before that time.

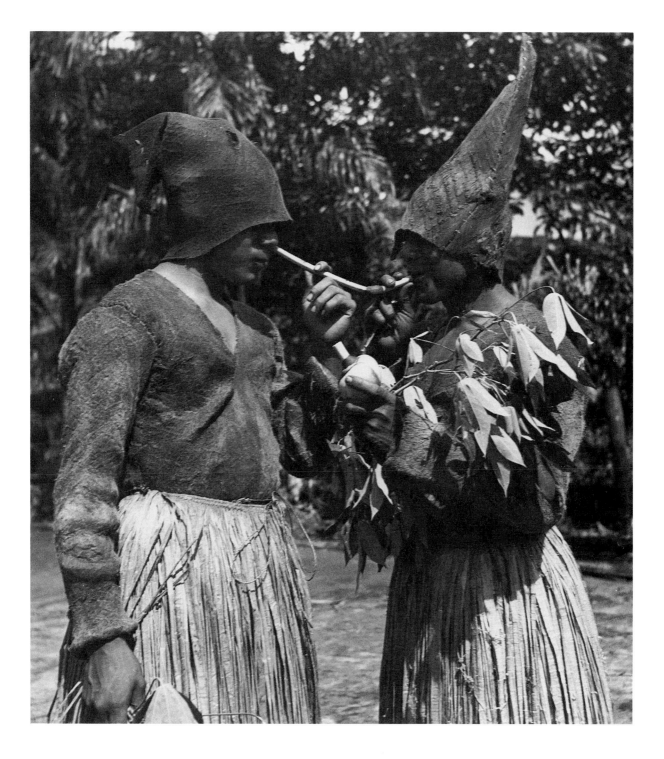

...for to make themselves drunke withall...

In the northwest Amazon, tobacco snuffing is frequently associated with Tukano-speaking Indians...Among the Barasana, neighbors of the Tukano, tobacco snuff features in their mythology.

J. Wilbert (1987)

# A famous Tanimuka payé self-administering snuff

*Caño Guacayá, Río Miritiparaná, Amazonas*

Tobacco snuff is an important aspect of the mythology amongst all tribes in the Colombian Amazonia, but particularly among the Tukanoans. To them, the payé increases his knowledge and understanding of the activity of the benevolent and malevolent spiritual forces with whom he must communicate during his seances. This photograph is of one of the famous medicine men of the Tanimukas who has adopted western dress but who still practises his profession with apparent great success.

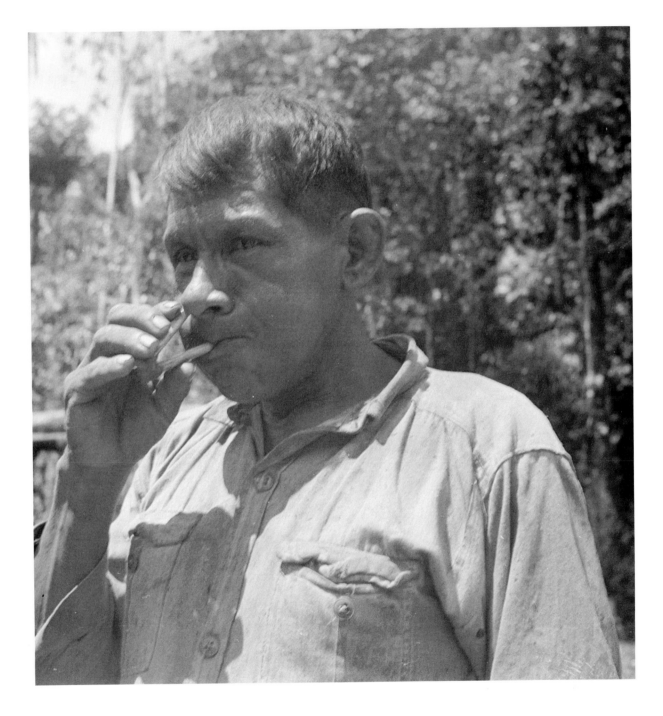

…snuff features in…mythology.

Tobacco is considered to be a ritual "non-food". It is...the food of the spirits.... Tobacco is believed to establish communication with the supernatural, and both snuff and tobacco smoke are said to have power;...

S. Hugh-Jones (1979)

# Yukuna youths taking snuff

*Caño Guacayá, Río Miritiparaná, Amazonas*

The widespread use of tobacco snuff is due in part to the belief amongst the Indians of the Colombian Amazon that it is a food of the spirits. As such, it "opens the mind" to an understanding of the wisdom of the spirit world. Snuff and tobacco in general, chewed or smoked, is believed to be a major medicine, a direct gift of the gods.

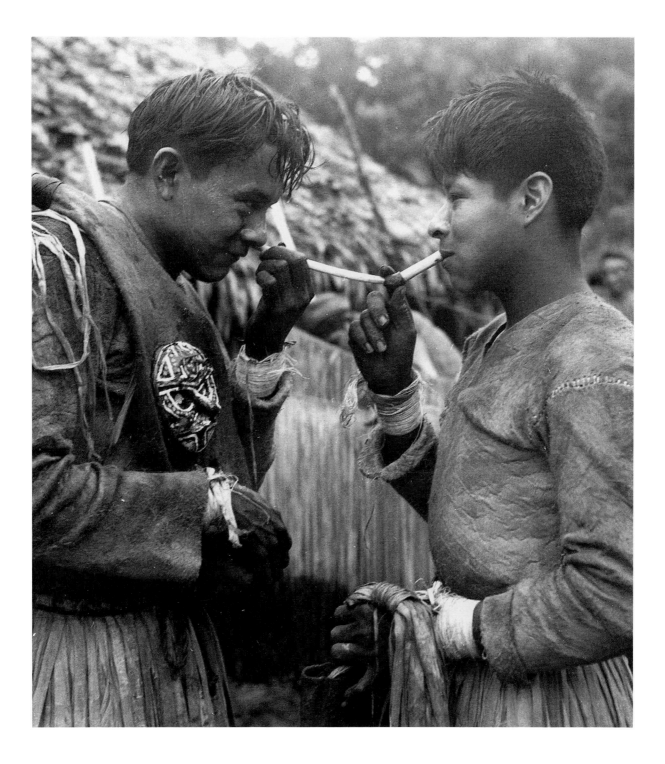

…food of the spirits…

These alkaline salts are prepared by evaporating water which has been poured over and drained through the ashes of various plants....

D. Kamen-Kaye (1971)

# Witoto apparatus for preparing alkaline "salt" for ambíl

*Arica, Río Putumayo, Putumayo*

The ashes of numerous plants may be used to obtain an alkaline residue formed following leaching the ashes with water and the final evaporation of the filtrate. Presumably, the inclusion of such "salts" in some of the Indians' plant preparations assists in the release of bioactive constituents from the plant materials.

The preferred source of the "salt" is the bark of the forest tree *Eschweilera itayensis*, but the stumps of terrestial and epiphytic species of numerous cyclanthaceous plants, particularly species of *Carludovica*, are frequently used in the same way.

Alkaline ashes or other alkaline plant products are employed nearly world-wide in alkaloidal preparations (coca, tobacco, betel nut, *Duboisia,* yopo, *Virola* snuff, etc.). It is of interest that societies in far-off regions have discovered that the presence of an alkaline substance actually facilitates the release of the narcotic or stimulating substance.

The method of preparation of the salt and the use are similar in the Colombian Amazon, and often the same plants are employed for preparing the ash with tobacco ambíl or with the coating of the hallucinogenic *Virola* pellets.

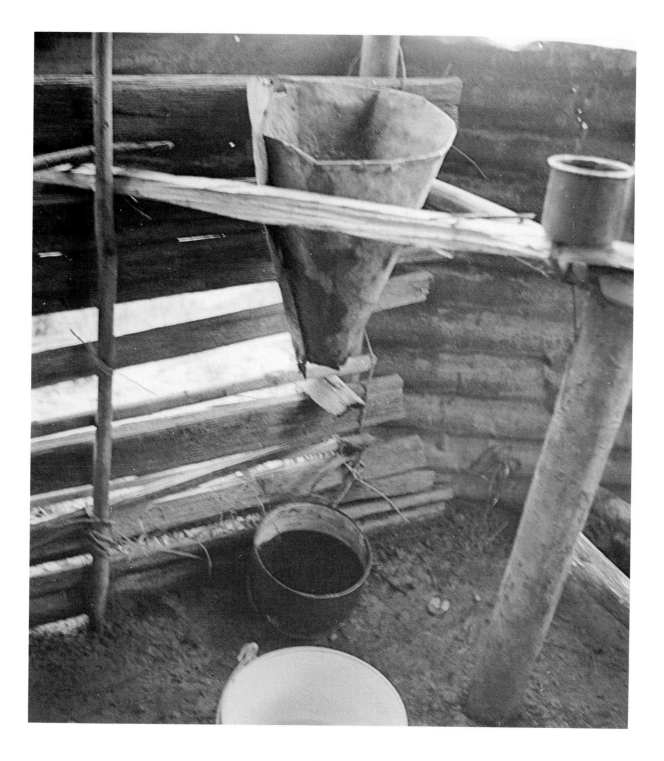

…alkaline salts are prepared…[from] various plants…

Upon the occasion of a fiesta or to solemnize any agreement or contract, they have recourse to the celebrated *chupé del tabaco* [tobacco sucking].... A numerous group of Indians congregate about a pot...which contains a strong extract of tobacco. The *capitán* [medicine man] first introduces the forefinger into the liquid and commences a long discourse.... Then they became more...excited, until finally the pot is gravely passed around, and each...dips his finger into the liquid and then applies it to the tongue. This is the Witoto's most solemn oath....

W.E. Hardenburg (1912)

# A Witoto taking ambíl from a cacao pot

*La Chorrera, Río Igaraparaná*

Tobacco syrup (ambíl) may be kept in a variety of containers, including an occasional glass bottle or a tin can, but the preferred container is made from a cacao shell which is said to add a sweet flavour to the syrup.

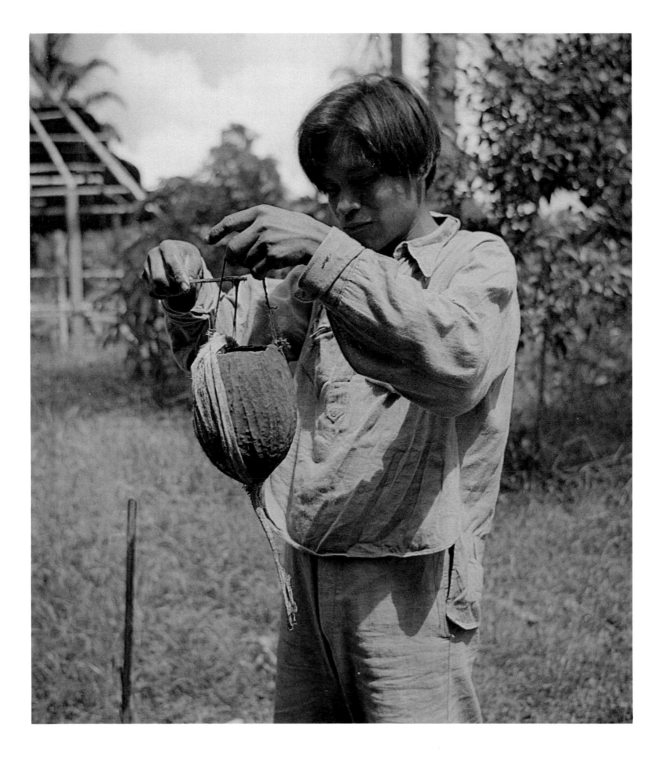

…the Witotos most solemn oath…

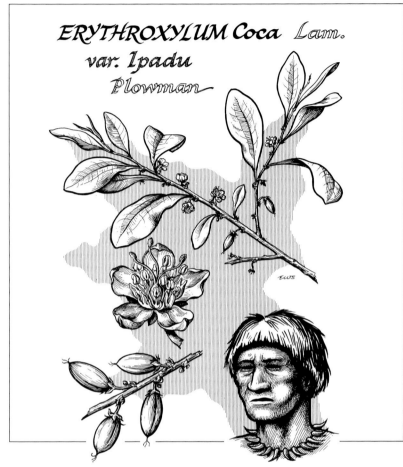

**ERYTHROXYLUM Coca Lam. var. Ipadu Plowman**

We now know that Amazonian coca belongs to the species *Erythroxylum Coca* but differs from the typical Andean species in a number of morphological and chemical features. I recently described Amazonian coca as a new variety named *Ipadú* after the common Brazilian name of [the plant].

T. Plowman (1981)

…Amazonian coca…differs from the typical Andean species…

## The Amazonian variety of *coca*

*Throughout the western Amazonia*

There is some disagreement concerning the age of the use of coca in the western Amazonia. Some opinions favour recent introduction from the Andean highlands. Others prefer to believe that its use is of great age in the region. First, it normally requires a considerable time for a new variety to develop; second, origin myths tell that the first settlers arrived in a dugout canoe dragged by an anaconda and bearing a man, a woman and three plants—manioc, yajé and coca; third, the coca plant is almost always planted in a plot separate from those used for food, thus signifying its special recognition as a sacred plant. These facts may be interpreted as suggestions of relatively great age of the use of this plant in the western Amazonia.

Darwin gave prominence to
the doctrine of Malthus that
organized life tends to increase
beyond the means of subsistence,
and emphasized a statement
of Spencer that...only the fittest
survive.... We have no more
pronounced example of these
laws than is illustrated in the
Coca plant. It has stood not only
the mere test of time but has
survived bitter persecution...

W.G. Mortimer (1901)

It has stood...the...test of
time...[and] has survived
...persecution.

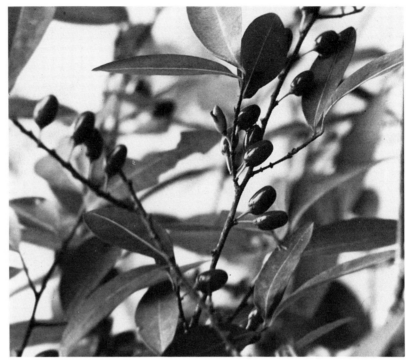

# The coca plant in fruit

*Río Kubiyú, Vaupés*

Coca has been persecuted from the earliest European arrival in South America and continues to be to this day as a result of the dangerous and illicit use of its principal bioactive constituent, cocaine, in many parts of the civilised world. The misuse of a chemically pure substance should not be confused with the "chewing" of coca leaves amongst Indians, particularly in the lowland regions, where it conceivably supplies certain elements lacking in the local diet.

Some of the healthiest and hardest working Indians of the Colombian Amazonia, the Yukunas, consume enormous amounts of coca leaves daily, but this is not a problem, as they have time to raise their crops, hunt, fish and supply their food. Coca chewing in the Andean highlands, by contrast, is a problem of poverty of the peasant miners and agriculturists who, working daily for overlords, have not the time to locate or raise enough food to assuage their hunger.

...coca is an integral part of the Indian's way of life, deeply involved with his traditions, his religion, his work and his medicine.

R.T. Martin (1970)

# A Makuna gathering coca leaves

*Río Piraparaná, Vaupés*

After a plot has been cleared for planting, most of the agricultural work in the Colombian Amazonia is done by women. There is, however, one exception. When coca leaves are to be gathered daily, it is only men and male youths who do the work. Once in the maloca, it may or may not be a woman who toasts the leaves, but it is always a man who pulverizes and sifts the powder and prepares the ashes for the final coca-ash mixture which is used.

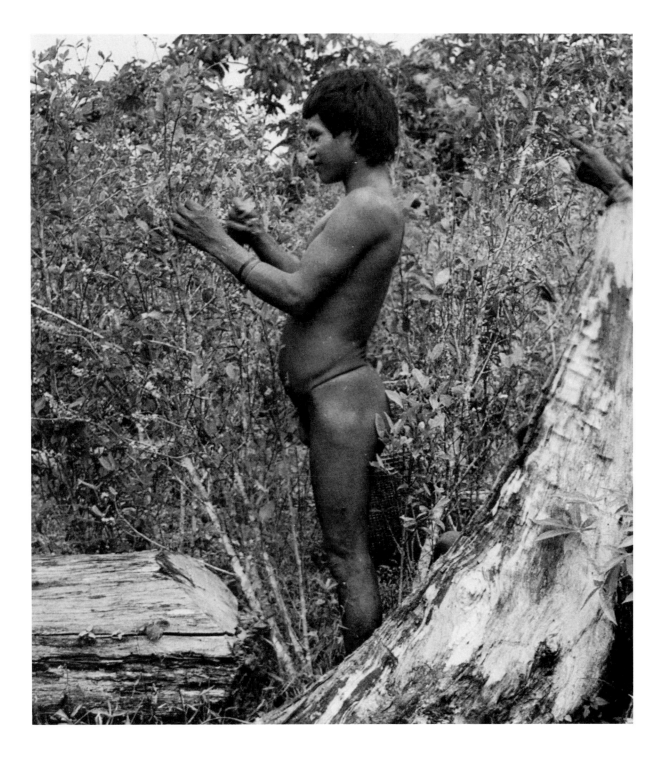

...an integral part...of life...

I found a small plantation of
ipadú [coca], a shrub of which
the powdered leaves are chewed
by the Indians...I found it to be
*Erythroxylon Coca*.

R. Spruce (1908)

## Koreguaje Indian with coca plant

*Nuevo Mundo, Caquetá*

Not all coca is produced by large stands of the plants. Many
Indians in the Colombian Amazonia live in small settlements at
the base of the Andes; the Koreguajes, for example, have a few
isolated plants for individual use near each house. Their consumption of the leaves is naturally much reduced from that of
most of the tribes living in the tropical lowland regions.

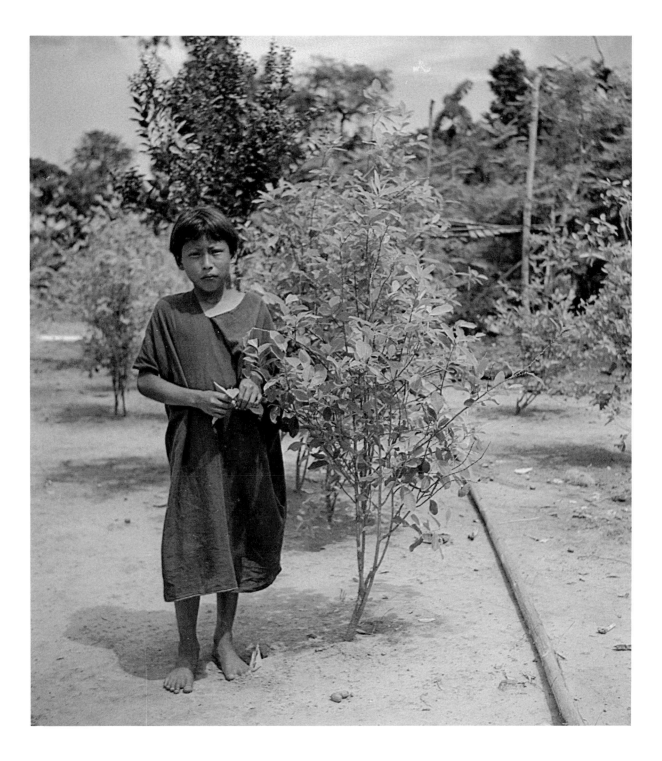

...a small plantation of *ipadú*...

After harvesting, the [coca] leaves
are carried in a woven basket
back to the communal maloca...
and immediately emptied into
a special coca toasting bowl or
manioc griddle over a slow fire
for drying.... This procedure may
take from 30 minutes...[or] to as
long as two hours...

T. Plowman (1981)

# Witoto toasting coca leaves

*La Chorrera, Río Igaraparaná, Amazonas*

The first operation following the collection of coca leaves during the afternoon is the toasting, as soon as possible, over a low round ceramic stone. This reduces the fresh leaves to a dry, brown material that is ready to be pulverized in a typical large mortar and pestle. Great care must be taken to avoid burning the leaves or subjecting them to too high a temperature.

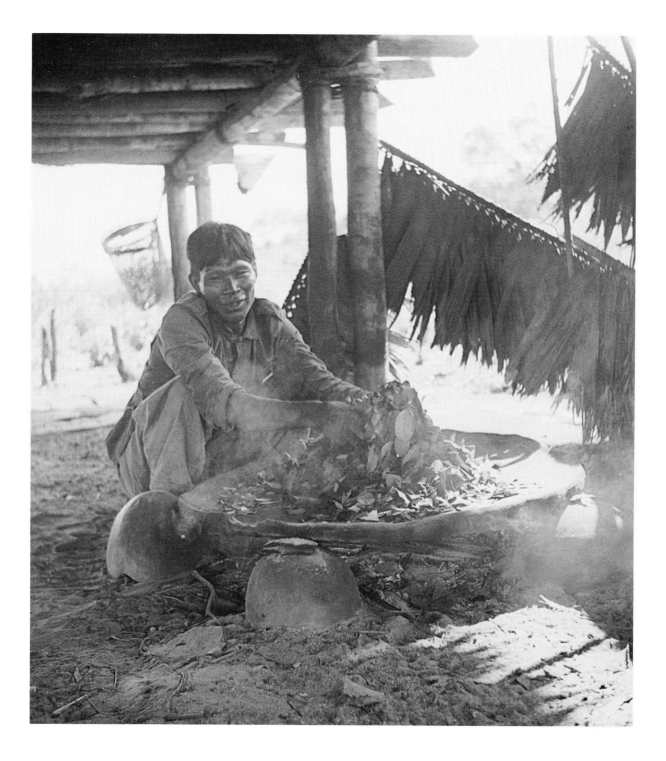

...leaves are emptied into a...coca bowl...for drying...

The method of preparation of Amazonian coca is remarkably similar throughout the upper Amazon, even among tribes that are linguistically unrelated and separated by great distances. The leaves are toasted and then pulverized.

T. Plowman (1981)

# Makuna payé pulverizing coca

*Río Piraparaná, Vaupés*

Coca leaves, as they are used in the northwest Amazon, are processed fresh each day: collected in the afternoon, toasted, then pulverized in a large mortar and mixed with the alkaline ash obtained usually by burning the *guarumo* tree (*Cecropia sciadophylla*). Early in the evening, the maloca resounds with the regular sound of the pestle, often accompanied by the chanting of a payé. It is one of the most enjoyable sounds the outside explorer encounters in his months of living in Indian malocas. Frequently the payé, or another knowledgeable tribal member will, during the preparation of the coca powder, recite tales of the mythology or origin of the race.

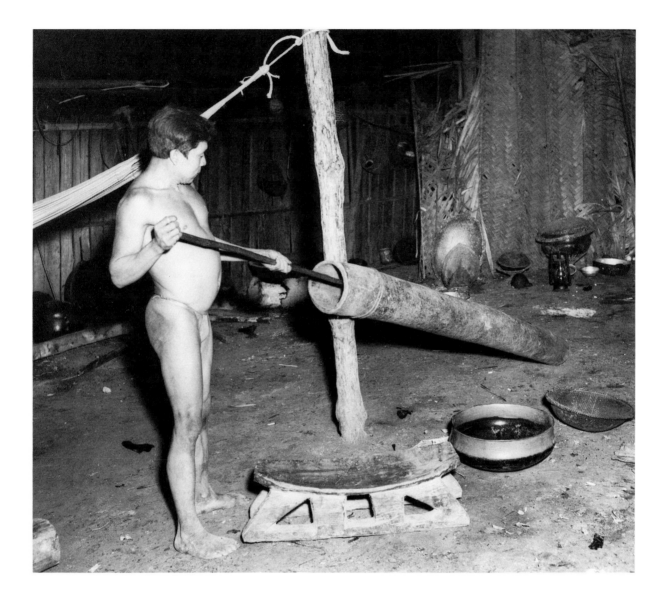

The leaves are…pulverized.

While coca is being pulverized, dead, fallen leaves of a species of Cecropia...which have been previously gathered and dried are burned to ashes. One of at least five species of Cecropia may be employed...,including *C. sciadophylla* Mart. Of these [this species] is preferred and the most widely utilized.

T. Plowman (1981)

# The best Cecropia for the ash admixture

*Mitú, Río Vaupés, Vaupés*

*Cecropia sciadophylla* of the Moraceae or Fig Family is a very tall tree which the Indians leave standing when they clear a piece of the forest for agriculture. Another moraceous tree, the leaves of which are frequently used for the same purpose, is the cultivated fruit tree *Pourouma cecropiaefolia* known locally as *uvilla* ("wild grape"). As the technical name indicates, the leaves of this plant are strikingly similar to those of *Cecropia*. The uvilla tree is close at hand, usually in the vicinity of the malocas.

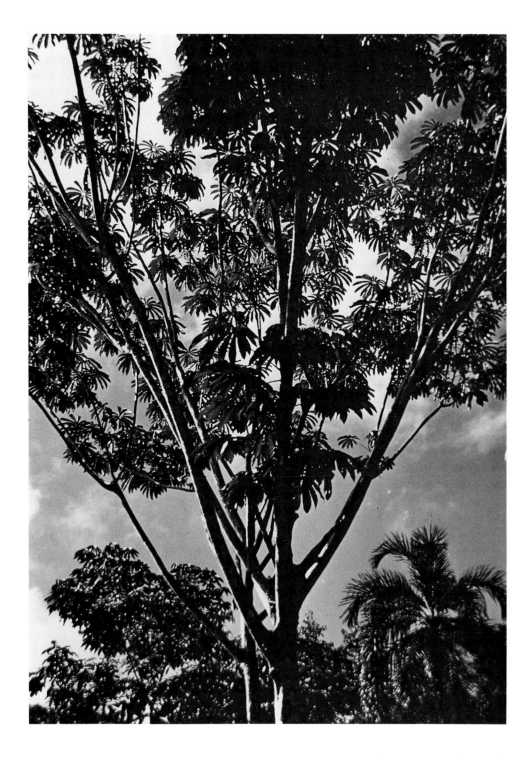

…leaves…are burned to ashes…

The Cecropia leaves are burned completely, leaving a fine whitish ash which is sifted once through a woven manioc strainer or, if very fine, after burning, simply added to the coca powder.

T. Plowman (1981)

# A Tanimuka preparing the ash admixture

*Río Kananarí, Vaupés*

Cecropia leaves are usually burned in the large central part of the malocas. When enormous quantities of coca must be prepared for the many guests invited to a tribal festival, the leaves are burned outside. There seems to be no reason for burning inside the houses, unless it be fear of rain. When the burning is carried on inside, the smoke does not interfere with normal Indian life, since the malocas are so constructed as to leave two large smoke holes at the peak of the roof which are referred to as "ears" in the native language.

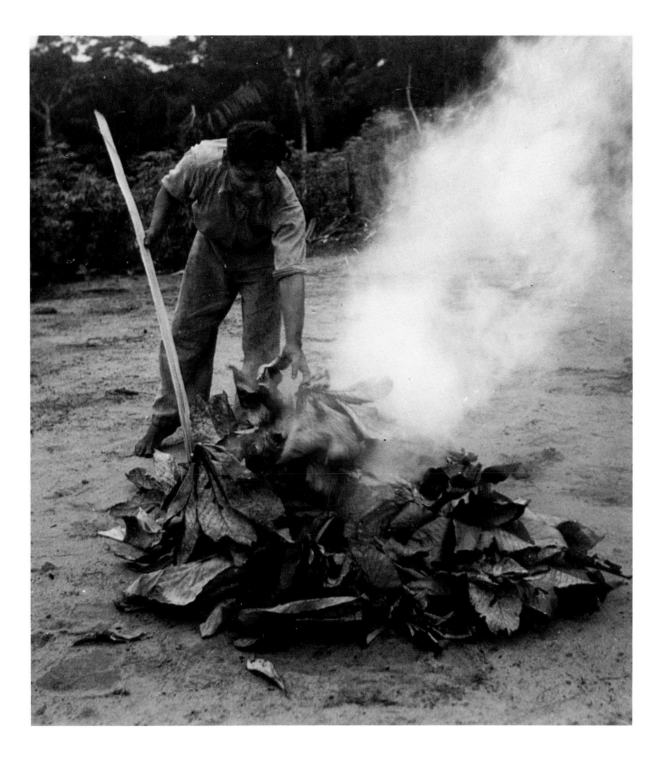

…Cecropia leaves are burned completely…

Perhaps the most ancient use of coca in South America is its employment in various shamanistic practices and religious rituals. As is the case with tobacco, the Indian medicine man valued coca specifically for its narcotic effects; the mild mental excitation... enabled him to enter more easily into a trance state in which he could communicate with the spiritual forces of nature and summon them to his aid.

R.T. Martin (1970)

# Barasana payé squeezing coca powder from a bark bag

*Río Piraparaná, Vaupés*

The usual method of putting powdered coca into the mouth employs a piece of leaf, a spoon prepared from a tapir bone or, often, a metal spoon. Some Indians of the Río Piraparaná have invented an ingenious apparatus, a bark-cloth bag fitted with a hollow bird bone spout. The drug is blown into the mouth by vigorously squeezing the bag which hangs during the day from a fibre belt that supports the loin cloth or *guayuco*. Not all Indian men take their coca in this way, but it appears to be favoured by most of the medicine men.

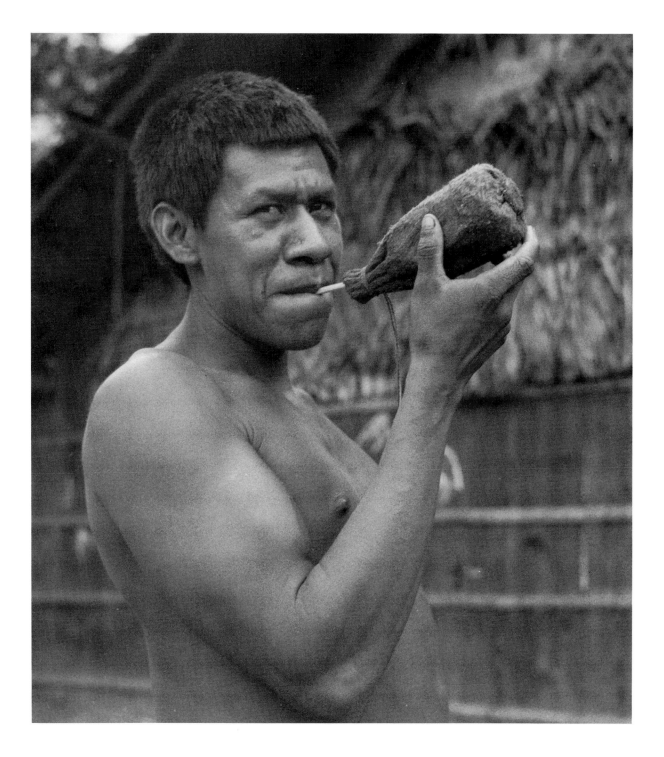

…to enter more easily into a trance state…

As with many plants used by the Indians of the western affluents of the Amazon...there seems to have been no knowledge of this species [*yoco*], the botanical identification of which was unknown, until a few years ago, although missionary reports mentioned it in the middle of the 18th Century.

V.M. Patiño (1967)

# A stimulant of the westernmost Amazon

*Colombian Putumayo and adjacent Ecuador*

Yoco (*Paullinia Yoco*, Sapindaceae) has been used for hundreds of years and was repeatedly reported in early Spanish missionary records. But until 1942, its botanical identity was not known. It is native only in the westernmost areas of the Amazonia in Colombia, Ecuador and Peru. With a high content of caffeine, it is the only plant the bark of which is the source of a stimulant caffeine drink: the beans or seed of coffee, *cola*, cacao, and *guaraná* are used, or the leaves of Chinese tea, *yerba maté, yaupon* and *guayusa*. Yoco bark yields about three percent of caffeine.

Yoco is an indispensable part of the diet of numerous Indian tribes in the area of its growth. The slow-growing forest liana is never cultivated. The plant is so extremely important in Indian economy that, when the wild sources near dwellings are depleted, the group simply moves on to a better location. With the exception of manioc, staff of life in this region, yoco is undoubtedly their most important plant, even though it supplies no real food.

114

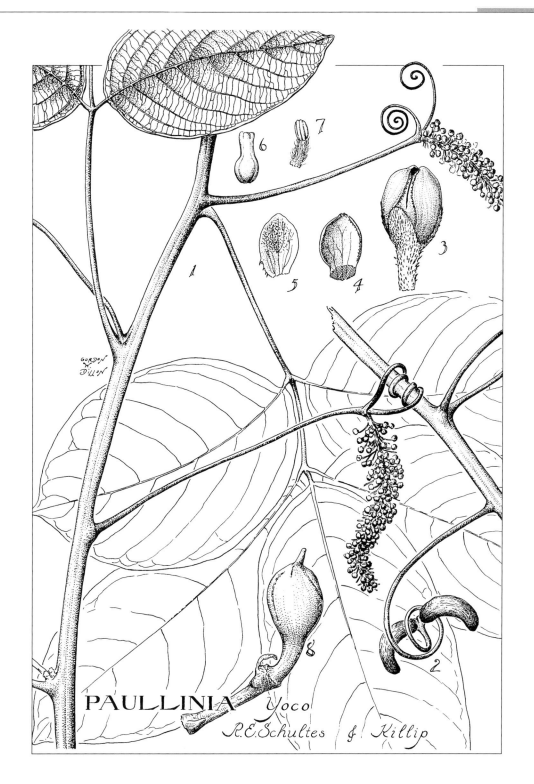

PAULLINIA *Yoco*
*R.E.Schultes & Killip*

…the botanical identification…was unknown, until a few years ago…

There is a *yoco blanco* ["white yoco"] and a *yoco colorado* ["red yoco"].

Zerda-Bayón (1906)

# Kofán rasping yoco

*Northwestern Amazonia*

The perspicacity of the Indians in noticing details is amazing. They often distinguish, and have names for, many "kinds" of a plant and frequently can identify them from a distance without touching, tasting or smelling them, even when a botanist cannot find any morphological differences and must consider them to represent a single species. In the case of yoco, for example, the Indians distinguish at least 15 "kinds". These types are well established in the Indian system of classification. This remains an enigma. Several explanations have been offered: soil or ecological conditions, chemical differences, age of the plants, the part of the plant taken, but all are conjectural and none satisfactorily explain the keeness of the Indian nor offer a "scientific" explanation for this phenomenon.

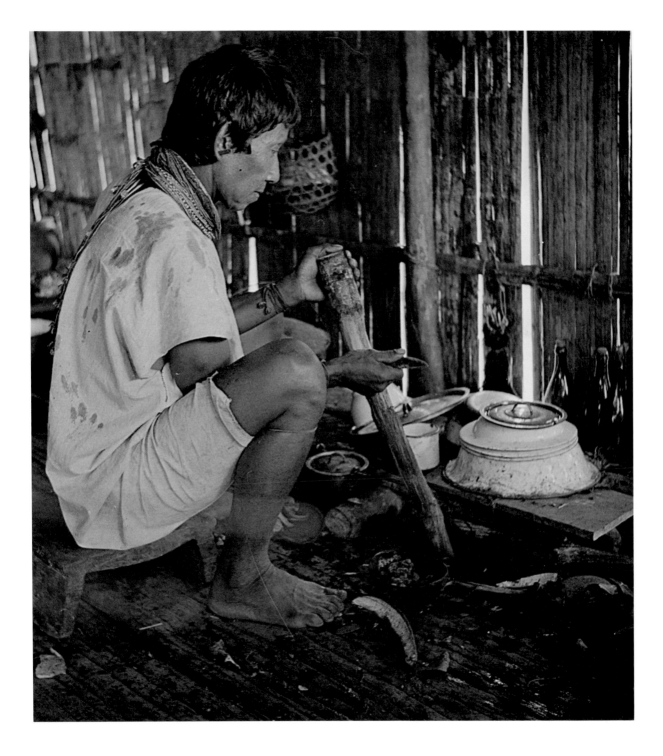

…a *yoco blanco* and a *yoco colorado*…

Yoco, their favourite beverage, is a liana, the bark of which in its green state is scraped off, kneaded and mashed in water and then thrown out. The remaining liquor assumes a yellowish brown...in general appearance.... Although the first taste is nauseating and bitter, the after-taste...is refreshing and not disagreeable. Yoco is imbibed at all hours; in the early morning much diluted and in larger quantity as an emetic..., and at times in stronger but smaller doses as a refreshment and sustenance.

A. Simson (1879)

## Kofán kneading the bark of yoco to prepare the drink

*Río Sucumbíos, Putumayo*

No food is normally taken in the early morning when, at 5:30 or 6:00 o'clock at the latest, the Indians awaken and rise. A gourdful of yoco is drunk, followed perhaps a half an hour later with another. If men expect to go hunting or fishing, they may even take more before leaving for the day. Pieces of the trunk of the extensive liana are kept in the malocas ready for use. When men embark on a canoe trip or long travel through the forest, pieces of the trunk are always carried. It is such a powerful stimulant that an Indian may go two days without food, sustaining himself on yoco.

It is usually a young man who is sent out to scout for a liana and collect it when a maloca needs to replenish its supply. A medicine man always accompanies the youth, and, before cutting down the liana and dividing it into yard-long pieces, he asks pardon for destroying such a "life giving" plant, and he assures the youth that he may safely destroy the vine.

118

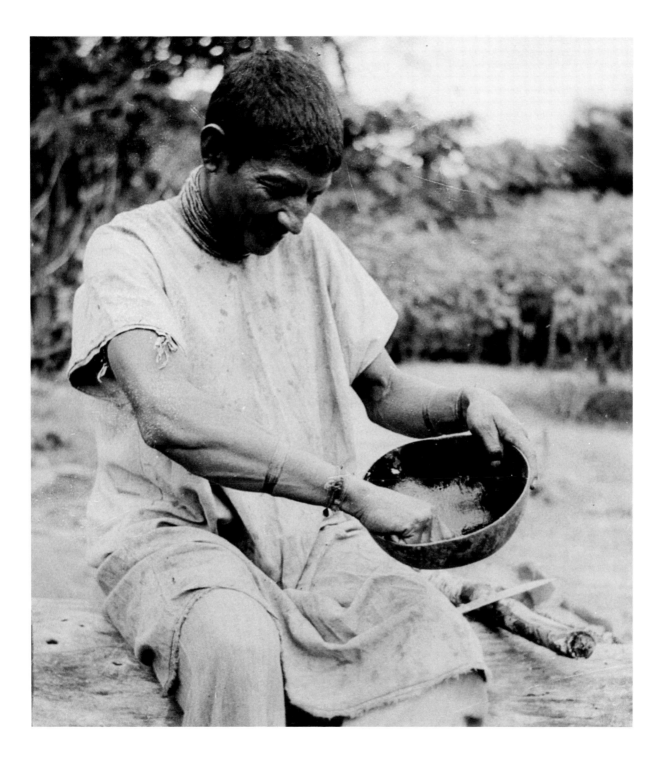

…the first taste is…bitter, the after-taste… refreshing…

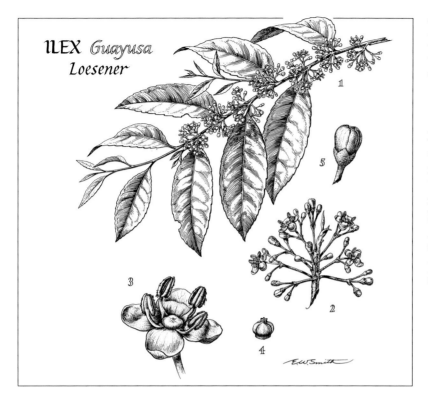

**ILEX** *Guayusa* Loesener

The guayusa is a true holly....
I was unable to find it in flower
or fruit and cannot say if it be a
described species.

R. Spruce (c. 1870)

In 1901, Theodore Loesener
described a new species of holly
from sterile material collected in
1898...in eastern Peru. Loesener
named the holly *Ilex Guayusa*
because the Indians of the
Amazonian Peru, Ecuador and
Colombia used its leaves to
prepare a medicinal beverage
tea called guayusa (or huayusa).

M. Shemluck (1979)

…guayusa…a true holly…

## The *guayusa* plant

*Northwesternmost Amazonia*

For many years—from the colonial days, when guayusa became
important commercially during the Spanish period to the present
time—the exact botanical identification of the source plant was
unclear. Only recently has this uncertainty been resolved with the
discovery of the rarely flowering shrub. It is now known that
guayusa is, as Spruce surmised over a century ago, a true holly, a
species of *Ilex*, a caffeine-containing plant.

The species was described from the specimens without flowers;
over 70 years elapsed before flowering material could be found.
The loss of flowering is frequently an indication of long cultivation of the plant.

There are two other species of *Ilex* valued as caffeine-containing
stimulants: I. *paraguariensis*, the yerba maté of Argentina, and I.
*vomitoria*, the yaupon of the southeastern part of the United States.

To maintain themselves at their best, they were accustomed to drink a decoction of an herb called guayusa...several times daily. They were thus able to stay awake without losing consciousness for many nights, when they feared an invasion by their enemies.

M. Jimínez de la Espada (1738)

To maintain themselves
at their best...

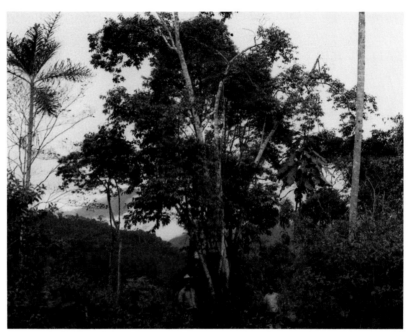

## Remnants of an ancient guayusa plantation

*Pueblo Viejo, Putumayo*

According to numerous missionary reports, there was great faith in the presumed medicinal value of guayusa, and a brisk export business of the leaves to Spain during the 17th century was developed. Extensive plantations of the tree were established to support the demand for this medicine, which was recommended for various illnesses but particularly as a cure for syphilis.

The leaves are still sold in the market places in Quito and Pasto. They are made into wreaths and sold by the wreath for medicinal use by the country people.

Guayusa was formerly employed over a greater area than it is today. The medicine men of Sibundoy and Mocoa in the Colombian Putumayo still value it highly as a cure-all. The tree is very rare in Colombia, but, following an early Jesuit report of "extensive plantations" in Pueblo Viejo near Mocoa, botanists have recently located 250 or 300 year-old trees in that remote and seldom-visited settlement. The trees are in excellent condition despite their age.

..they use the juice of a...tree they call *solyman*.... The effect of the juice seems to be restricted to the breathing apparatus of the fish, which rise to the surface... gasping for air, where they may easily be caught...

G. MacCreagh (1926)

# A useful but mysterious tree

*Río Vaupés*

This mysterious small tree or shrub has been put to local use in at least two ways. It is not only a fish poison, but the bark provides a method of temporary tattooing.

The crushed leaves of *Duroia hirsuta* (Rubiaceae), thrown into still water, affect the breathing apparatus of fish, forcing them to come to the surface for oxygen.

It is also used in a ceremonial or superstitious connection. The Indians bind around the arms and legs a strip of fresh bark with the inner surface touching the skin. The strips are removed after several hours, leaving water blisters. In a day or so, the blisters disappear, and a blue-black mark, which lasts a month or more, remains. The caustic constituent has apparently not been chemically identified.

The shrub is also feared and respected as the sole arborescent inhabitant of strange, cleared areas in the forest called "Gardens of the Devil".

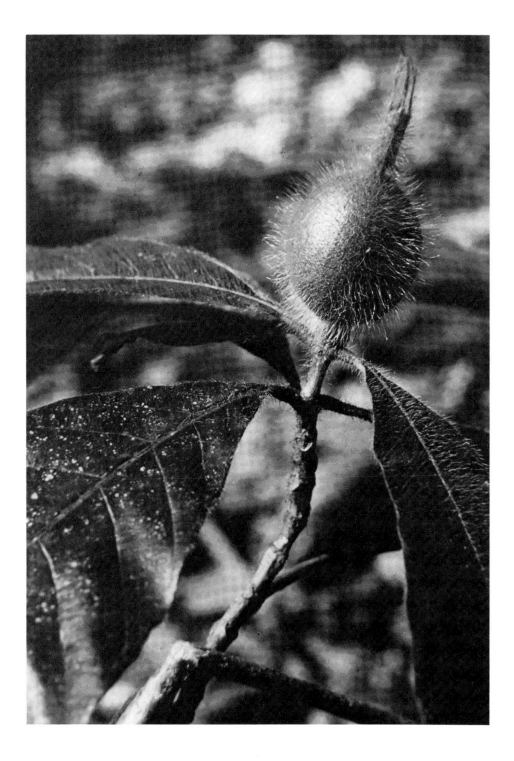

...the juice of *solymán*...

Numerous tribes...cannot bear
the taste of salt, but tribes which
do enjoy it use native salt, bitter
as it is, in large quantities.

C. Lévi-Strauss (1950)

# A river weed on rocks

*Falls of Jerijerimo, Río Apaporis, Vaupés*

The Vaupés Indians are very fond of our table salt; and, whenever
they can get it, they eat it by the tablespoonful.

However, the very abundant river weed *Rhyncholacis nobilis*
(Podostemonaceae) growing profusely on all the rapids of the Río
Apaporis and Vaupés, is gathered, dried and burned to provide
their substitute for sodium chloride which, of course, is not
available.

The plant is widely known as carurú and is used over a wide area
of the northwest Amazon as a source of salt for use with food.

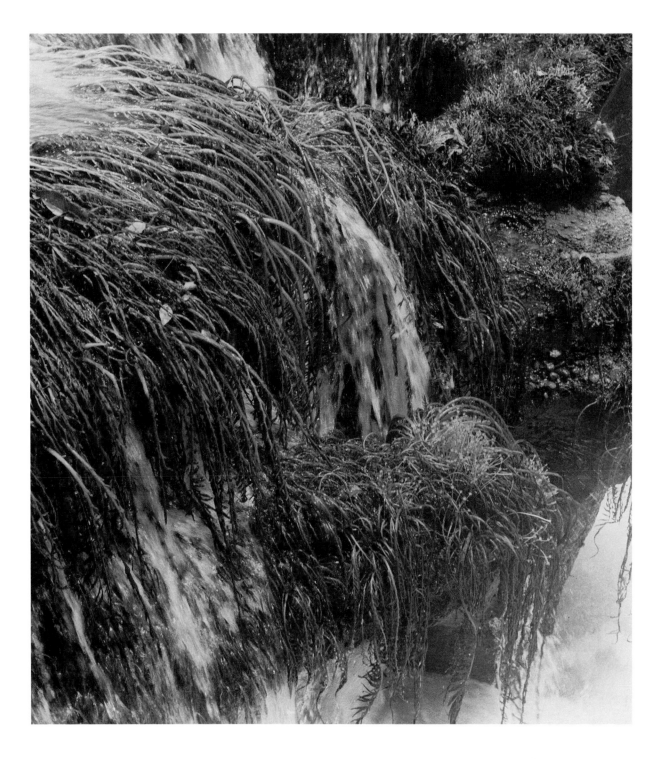

native salt…in large quantities.

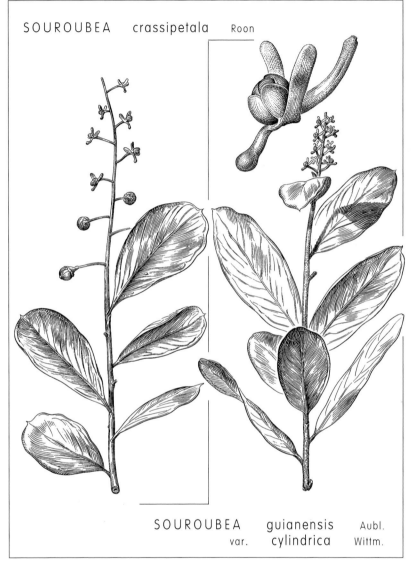

SOUROUBEA   crassipetala   Roon

SOUROUBEA   guianensis   Aubl.
var.   cylindrica   Wittm.

...artificially induced sleep among the Indians is one of their bits of portentious witchery.

R. Gill (1940)

...induced sleep [and] witchery.

# Two sleep-inducing plants

*Río Apaporis, Vaupés*

Medicine men in the northwest Amazon often suggest sleep as a remedy, especially amongst the aged and those patients experiencing psychological problems. The payés have knowledge of a number of plants to prescribe for inducing sleep; the two most commonly used are species of Souroubea of the Marcgraviaceae.

The *manioc* gardens are essentially the domain of the women, but the men plant coca, tobacco, fish-poisons and yajé...and make almost daily visits to pick coca leaves.

S. Hugh-Jones (1979)

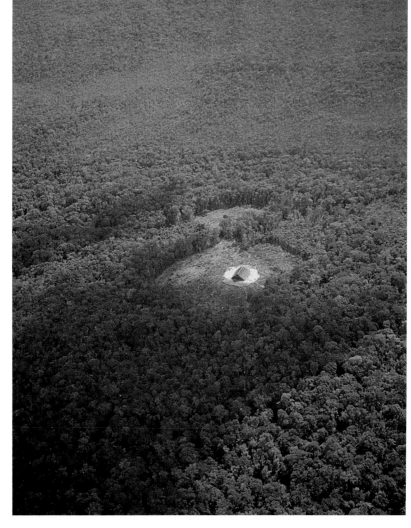

...manioc gardens are...
the domain of...women,
...men plant coca...

## *Manioc* and coca in separate plots

*Río Piraparaná, Vaupés*

In most tribes, agriculture is practiced in two separated plots. Manioc and other food sources are planted and tended wholly by the women, and the manioc garden is usually near the maloca. In a second plot, often quite a distance away, plants of a sacred or ceremonial importance are cared for exclusively by the men. Both plots are chosen, as are house sites, after consultation with a local payé.

The amount of time it takes for a festival to be prepared depends on the amount of *chicha* to be consumed. With over a hundred people..., four days were barely enough for the manioc roots to be rubbed down, the poisonous juice extracted and then boiled to form the basis of chicha.... The boiling liquid was poured into the long chicha canoe.... The chicha gained rapidly in potency.

B. Moser and D. Tayler (1965)

# An essential element in every dance

*Río Loretoyacu, Amazonas*

*Chicha*, a slightly fermented drink made usually from manioc but occasionally from various fruits—pineapple, bananas, cananguche and others—is an absolute essential in great quantities for ceremonial or even ordinary dances. It is prepared usually in long dugout canoes, and guests and participants are free to dip a gourd into the liquid and drink freely throughout the length of the festival which may last for several days with fifty or a hundred or more adult attendants.

The women must work for at least 10 days preparing enough manioc root to allow it to ferment before the day of arrival of the guests.

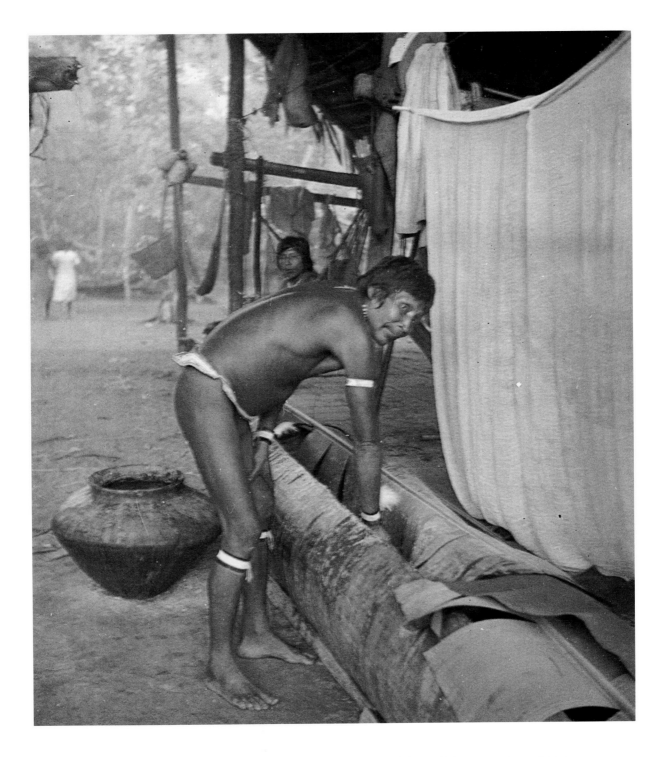

The chicha gained rapidly in potency.

Since it was the manioc festival, only the ceremonial *Nahuabasa* —signifying the complete cycle of manioc from the time it was planted to the time it became cassava—was danced...The manioc dance continued through the night.... Throughout the entire festival, the dominating figure was the shaman.... It was he who influenced the festival which, without him, would not take place. Every few hours, he summoned the elders...and, as coca was passed round, the mysterious chanting began.

B. Moser and D. Tayler (1965)

## Preparation of manioc bread for festival

*Araracuara, Río Caquetá, Amazonas*

The manioc plant is the principal food of all Indians of the Amazon, almost their sole source of carbohydrate.

There are two strains of the euphorbiaceous *Manihot esculenta*; one with a high concentration of a toxic cyanogenetic glycoside present throughout the root, one with a low concentration localized primarily in the bark of the root. It is the former strain that is almost exclusively cultivated in the Amazon.

As the staff of life, manioc is accorded an important role in ritual and ceremonial dances, in origin myths and in the various circumscriptive shamanistic controls on choice of agricultural sites, felling of the forest, planting and harvesting and preparation of manioc flour.

Enormous quantities of manioc flour *[cassava]* and *chicha* must be prepared for all of the heavily attended tribal ceremonies and dances.

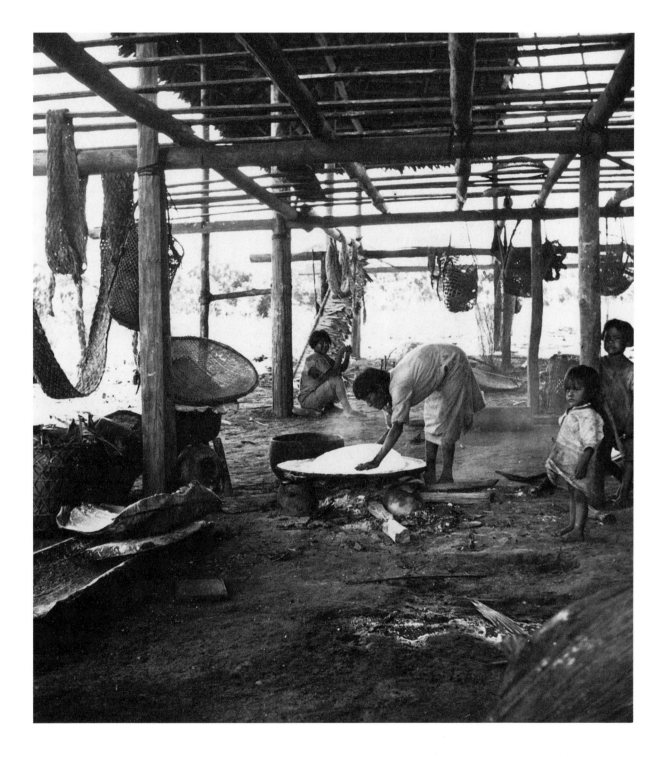

the manioc festival...signifying [the transformation of] manioc...[to] cassava...

Chicha, an intoxicating drink...,
is supposedly purifying and
ritualistic.

D. Stone (1948)

# Kubeo imbibing chicha

*Río Kuduyarí, Vaupés*

The alcoholic content of chicha is low, but intoxication is invariably induced. The Indian, however, looks upon intoxication as a religious state; during an intense intoxication, whether from alcoholic drinks or hallucinogenic drugs, the soul leaves the body to wander in far off supernatural realms. The disappearance of the symptoms of intoxication signifies the return of the soul to the body.

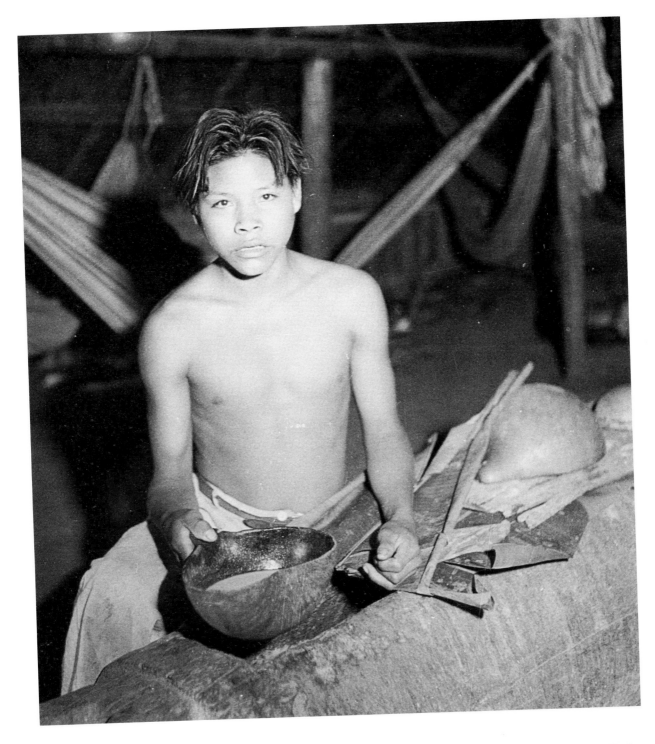

...purifying and ritualistic.

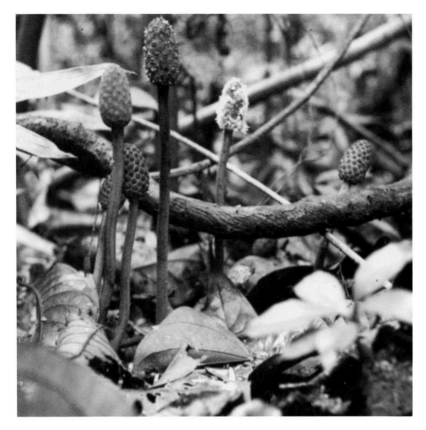

Damp shady hollows, where the vegetable mould lay deep, were often overspread with *Helosis brasiliensis* Mart. [of the Balanophoraceae], one of the lowest forms of flowering plants, looking quite like the young state of some fungus...until what seems to be an unexpanded cap is found to be a solid oval head of reddish brown colour, studded with minute flowers of the most rudimentary structure.

R. Spruce (1908)

...like the young state of some fungus...

## A strange species of the Amazonian flora

*Río Loretoyacu, Amazonas*

Known in Colombia as *cojamba*, this curious blood-red obligate parasite that grows on the roots of trees and shrubs is valued by Indians in the Vaupés and Amazonas as an effective medicine, *Heliosis guyannensis* (Balanophoraceae). Dried and pulverized, it is a strong astringent and is said to be an excellent styptic; it is also taken in a decoction for treating dysentery and diarrhea.

Medicine men are said to hold it in high esteem, but whether as a medicine because of its queer method of growth or as a result of its blood-red colour which seems to be of special shamanistic significance, is not known.

Is it possible that its colour of blood first suggested its native use as a styptic?

134

We find in the Apocynaceae numerous properties.... In general, they are bitter, stimulating and slightly astringent;...when these properties are weak, they may be useful, whilst when they are present to excess, they may become dangerously toxic.

P. LeCointe (1934)

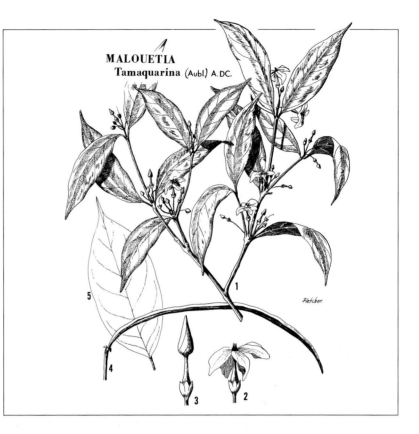

MALOUETIA
Tamaquarina (Aubl) A. DC.

...they may be useful, whilst... (in) excess they may become...toxic

# A toxic but useful plant

*Mitú, Río Vaupés, Vaupés*

This common riparian plant is known in Spanish as *cuchara-caspi* ("spoon tree") because the Indians carve spoons from its soft wood. It is usually infested with hordes of ferocious ants. *Malouetia Tamaquarina* has highly poisonous leaves; but this toxicity notwithstanding, they are added to the hallucinogenic drink, caapi, by Makuna medicine men of the Río Popeyaká. The latex has been employed as an ingredient of a type of curare and is painted on wounds to hasten healing.

According to natives of the Río Loretoyacu who enjoy the flesh of the *pajuíl* bird as food, the bird eats the fruit of this small tree. The bones of the pajuíl must not be fed to dogs during the fruiting of cuchara-caspi, lest they poison the dogs, causing immediate and violent gastric upset, a glassy-eyed stare, lack of muscular coordination and frequently death.

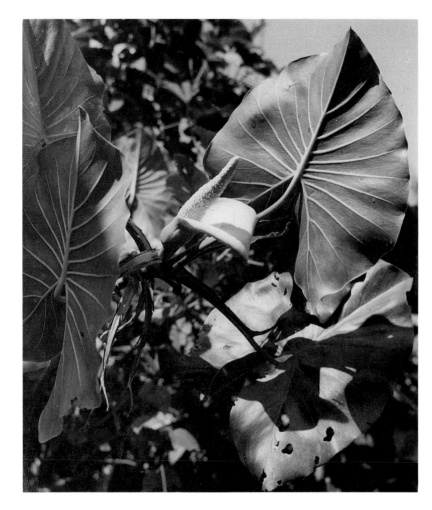

Some form of magic or ritual is performed in every society with the hope of influencing the outcome of events. Aroids have had an important part to play in several different cultures.

D. Bown (1988)

...influencing the outcome of events.

## A gigantic Amazonian aroid

*Leticia, Río Amazonas, Amazonas*

This arborescent aroid, *Montrichardia arborescens* (Araceae), grows in incredible abundance along the floodable banks of the Río Amazonas. Tikuna medicine men in the Río Loretoyacu near Leticia report that, whenever a difficult case appears for their decision, they gather the leaves of this plant, dry and pulverize them. The powder is blown widely over those who are gathered for the shamans' decision in the belief that this can help them arrive at a correct diagnosis. There is, as yet, no explanation for this use, inasmuch as no active chemical has been reported from the plant.

Birthworts [*Aristolochiae*] are notable for their thick bark cloven down to the woody axis in six or more furrows. When cut across, they give out a strong smell, usually rather fetid, but in some cases pleasantly aromatic. They are scarce in the...Amazon valley, and their singular hooded and often lurid-coloured flowers are difficult to find.

R. Spruce (1908)

ARISTOLOCHIA
medicinalis
R.E. Schultes

...they are scarce in the Amazon valley...

## A favourite medicine of the payés

*Urania, Río Vaupés, Vaupés*

The astringent root, dried and powdered, is prescribed by Kubeo medicine men for periodic attacks that appear to be of an epileptic nature. According to the Indians, it is dangerous and must be used sparingly as it may, in heavy doses, cause permanent metal disorders or muscular paralysis.

Species of Aristolochia are not frequent in the Amazon flora; their curious hooded and colourful flowers may be partly responsible for the native belief in their medicinal activity. The genus does, however, have interesting chemical constituents, which we are only recently beginning to investigate in tropical species.

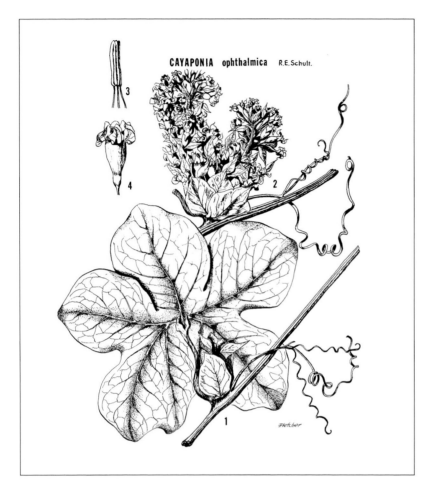

CAYAPONIA ophthalmica  R.E.Schult.

Conjunctivitis [or] inflammation of the conjunctiva, the mucous membrane covering the eyeball and the inner part of the eyelids …is caused by bacteria. The eye becomes pink from inflammation, hence the condition is also called pinkeye. This is very contagious [but] can usually be cured by simple home treatment.

Readers Digest
Health Guide (1970)

…unusually cured
by simple…treatment

# A medicine for eye infections

*Río Popeyaká, Amazonas*

One of the most common diseases of the Amazon is conjunctivitis. It frequently attacks many or all of the people living in the large communal *malocas*, as it is highly contagious. The children seem to be more frequently infected than the adults. Of the several plants used against this condition, the one said by the Indians of the Vaupés to be most effective, is a vine of the Gourd Family, *Cayaponia ophthalmica*, which is cultivated for this purpose by the medicine men.

The leaves are boiled gently, and the tea is dropped onto the affected area over a period of three or four days.

A common illness,...*susto* is an intense psychic trauma provoked by an emotion of fear and includes lack of appetite and energy. Susto is caused by the loss of the sick person's soul.

M. Dobkin de Rios (1973)

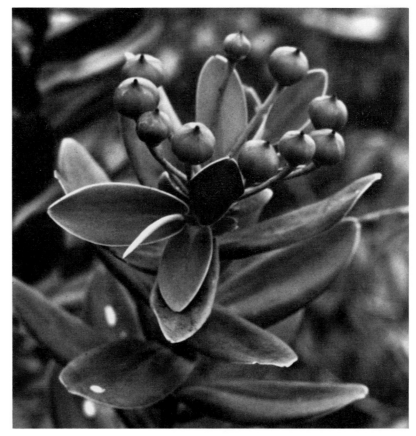

...loss of the sick person's soul.

## A tranquilizer valuable to treat *susto*

*Río Piraparaná, Vaupés*

The number of people—particularly women and children—who suffer attacks of susto is amazing. The word means "fright" in Spanish, but susto is the result of a psychological fright or disequilibrium brought on by fear of punishment or death from supernatural sources. It is thought that psychological maladjustment can be cured only with psychological methods, although many biologically oriented psychiatrists do not agree. The medicine men, however, usually employ a combination of psychical and medical treatment, and they have several tranquilizing plants that they prescribe together with their incantations and reliance on superstitions. One of the plants considered most successful is *Souroubea guianensis* var. *cylindrica* (Marcgraviaceae), an abundant low shrub primarily of the margins of xerophytic savannahs.

Few primitive people have acquired as complete knowledge of the physical and chemical properties of their botanical environment as the South American Indian.... it is probable that only a fraction of the herbs used by modern Indians are presently known and exploited.

C. Lévi-Strauss (1950)

# A Kubeo panacea

*Urania, Río Vaupés, Vaupés*

From two payés and ordinary Kubeo natives, *Mandevilla Steyermarkii* (Apocynaceae) an unusual plant was indicated to be effective for a wide spectrum of medicinal uses. The Kubeo name, *da-pá-kö-da* indicates its medicinal fame: *da* signifies a medicine, and it appears twice in the name.

The latex is considered a help in healing sores and skin infections when painted on the area. When toasted and powdered, the leaves are added to *chivé* (a watery porridge of manioc flour) to stem diarrhea. The flowers are soaked in chicha to lend presumed aphrodisiac properties to the fermented drink during the famous Yurupari ceremony. Chewing the highly laticiferous stem is said to relieve bleeding from the gums. One elderly payé maintained that a tea of the bark of the lower part of the stem was efficacious in preventing whitening or loss of hair. Another payé insisted that the plant is "poisonous" and must not be used without consultation with the medicine men. He also maintained that this is one of the few plants that are "dangerous to employ", because it was a gift of the spirits.

Our preliminary chemical field tests on this interesting climber indicated that it did not contain alkaloids. Its fame as a medicine and its alleged spiritual origin may be in great part the result of the unusual floral form and colouration and its endemic rarity more than any actual bioactive properties.

The plant is rare, known only from southern Venezuela and the Colombian Vaupés.

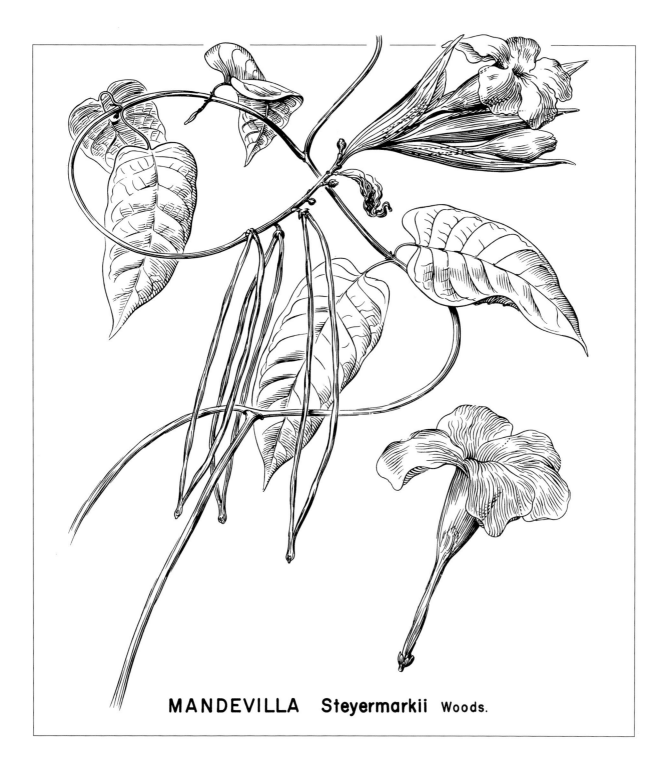

**MANDEVILLA Steyermarkii Woods.**

...a fraction of the herbs used...are known and exploited...

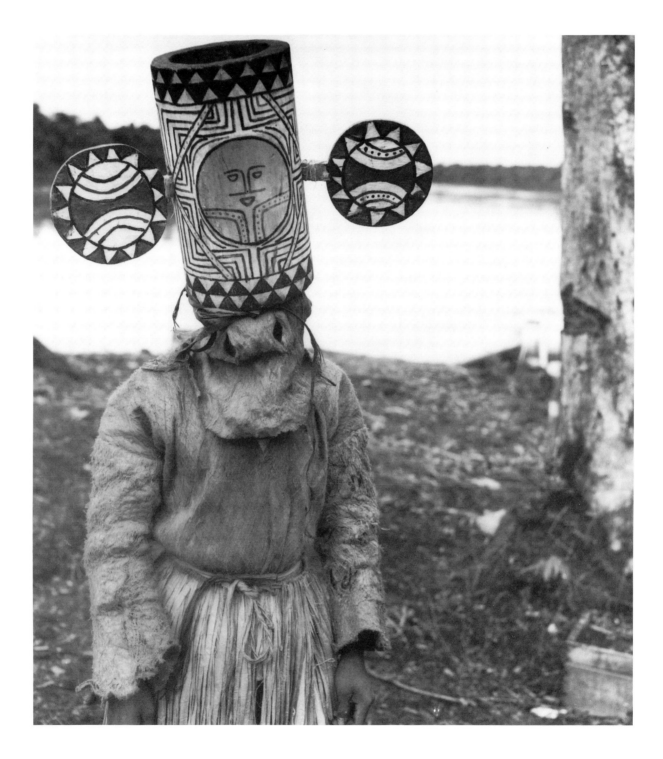

The Sun created the…principle of good…and evil…

The Sun created the universe
and...he is called Sun-Father....
The Sun created the animals and
plants.... the Sun created the night
people and put them in the dark
region.... To them he gave the job
of serving as intermediaries for
witchcraft and sorcery, because
the Sun did not only create the
principle of good but also of evil
to punish mankind when it did
not follow the customs of tradition.

G. Reichel-Dolmatoff (1971)

## Balsa-wood sun mask for the *Kai-ya-ree* dance

*Río Miritiparaná, Amazonas*

Since the Kai-ya-ree is basically a religious ceremony to plead for
favourable treatment from the forces of darkness, the Wagti, it
seems to the natives obligatory to try to propitiate the forces of
light, the sun, which in reality makes life possible on earth. Like
Wagti, the Sun could act for both good and evil, and through the
inflicting of eclipses and unfavourable seasons, floods and other
climatic misfortunes, he could punish mankind for not living
according to prescribed ways.

The large cylindrical balsa-wood mask that is worn on the head
of the dancers taking part in the fourth day of the Kai-ya-ree
dances, has painted, in yellow mineral colouring, the image of the
sun. It is the dance in which only adult males and the payés
themselves may participate—indicative of the great importance
of this specific dance for the future safe-guarding of the welfare
of the tribe.

The shamans can even enclose themselves in a bubble of air and so enter the sacred waterfalls and descend to the river bed, where they negotiate for days on end with the Master of the Fish.

F. Trupp (1981)

## The Falls of Jerijerimo, sacred to the Taiwanos

*Río Apaporis, Vaupés*

This and similar "achievements" of payés—such as their ability to turn into jaguars at will—are unquestionably accepted by the Indians who look upon the powerful members of the tribes as exceptional individuals set aside from ordinary men by supernatural forces that make it possible to accomplish what cannot be explained by normal human activity. It is usually through the various hallucinations that shamans are able, the Indian believes, to transcend everyday life and transfer themselves to unworldly regions.

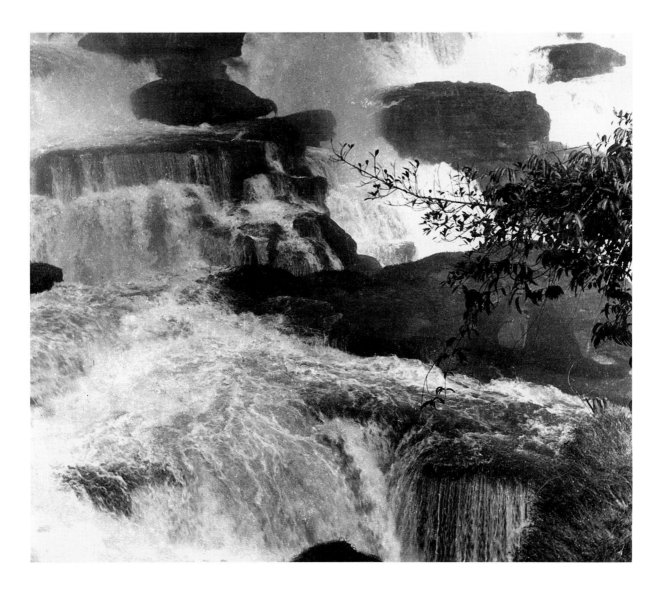

The shamans can…enter the sacred waterfalls…

When in 1820...Martius caught sight of the Cerro de Cupatí (now called La Pedrera) following several wearisome months paddling upstream in the Amazon and Caquetá rivers, he felt that he was entering a different world. Here, the crushing monotony of the flat Amazonian forest is broken and one's vision rests with the contrast that is presented by this small undulation of the landscape of 150 meters—like an island in the midst of an intensely green ocean. The great scientist sensed the bewitchment of the "Sacred Mountain" two days before arriving, when he saw it for the first time from his slow canoe, paddled by Indians.

C.A. Domínguez (1987)

# A fantastic monument to Nature

*Cerro de La Pedrera, Río Caquetá, Amazonas*

Located on the Río Caquetá a few miles above the mouth of the Río Apaporis, this picturesque mountain is not only sacred to the Mirañas but harbours many endemic plants not known from any other locality. It was first collected by the famous German botanist von Martius and, the work of several more recent plant explorers notwithstanding, some of the species that he discovered and described have not been recollected. One of the local payés realizes this high endemism and attributes it to supernatural interest in this mountain. Its flora has not yet been systematically studied, and it has been suggested that the mountain should be protected as a biological reserve in view of its great importance to science.

146

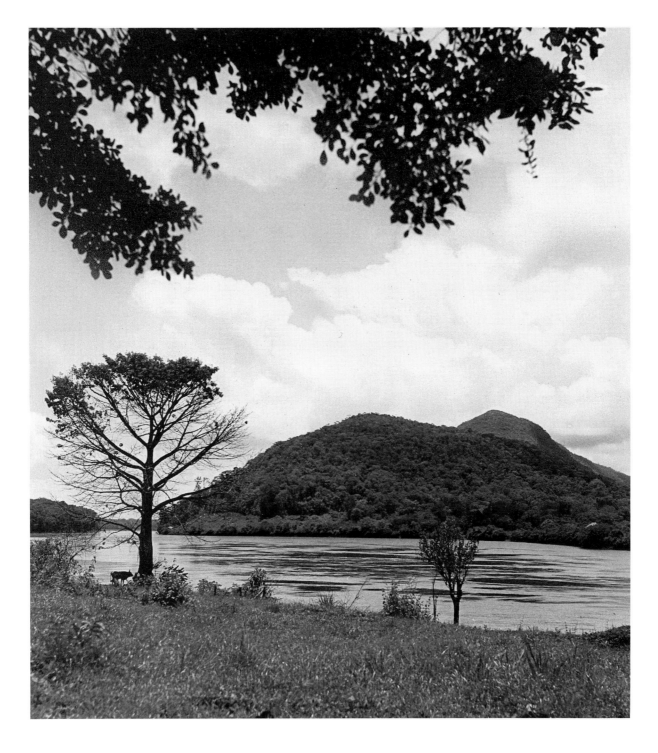

…an island in the midst of an intensely green ocean.

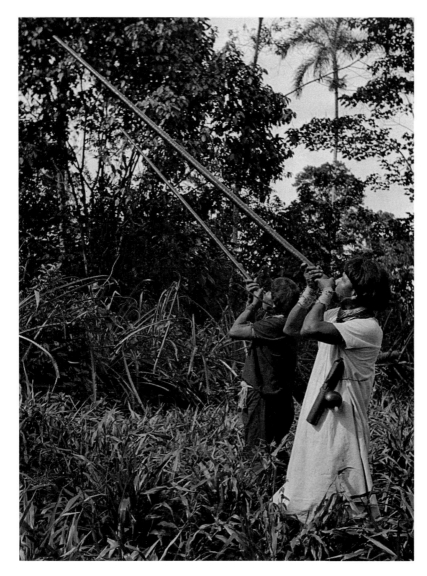

Before the Indians go hunting, they have to observe certain rituals, because the act of killing a wild animal is otherwise considered evil...the payé... appeals to...the Master of Animals for permission for the Indians to hunt and kill game. If they fail to consult the spirit, they must expect...[the spirit] to avenge the offence...by sending illness or poisonous snakes or by calling tornadoes to devastate their homes and crops.

F. Trupp (1981)

...the payé appeals... for permission for the Indians to hunt....

## Siona Indians shooting monkeys for food

*Mocoa, Putumayo*

Monkeys are often prevalent along the edges of jungle forest where it is easier to shoot them. Why this should be is difficult to explain, since monkeys tend to live in the densest forests. They may prefer nearness to human habitation. But it is well known that hunters prefer to practise their skills or to test new blowguns in the vicinity of forest clearings.

The traditional attitude toward drink and intoxication is religious, not secular. They do not drink for mere pleasure or to overcome anxiety. Secular drinking is for them distasteful, and it is rare to see an [unacculturated] Indian drunk except at a ceremony.

I. Goldman (1963)

...intoxication is religious, not secular.

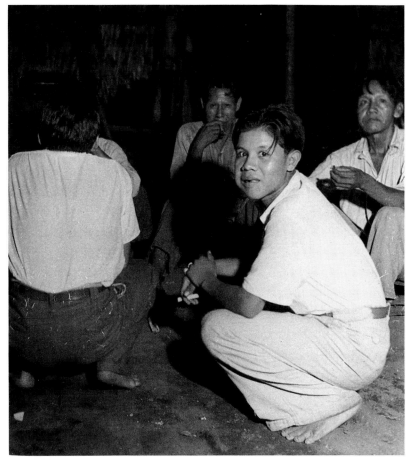

## Kubeos in an evening conversation drinking chicha and chewing coca

*Río Kuduyarí, Vaupés*

Since the Indian population of the Colombian Amazon has no distilled liquor until it is brought in from the outside, the consumption of alcohol is in the form of fermented chicha prepared from *yuca* or various fruits. The alcoholic content is low, and the intoxication produced rarely leads to bellicosity.

Many evening "get togethers", when stories are shared by half a dozen friends or when a payé recites the mythological tales of the tribes' origin and history, are enlivened by social use of chicha or coca.

149

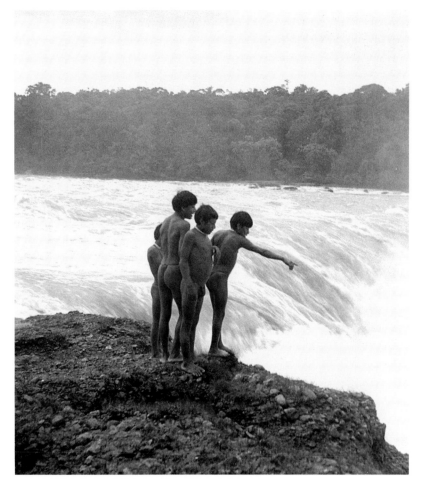

To the natives of the Vaupés...the rivers and their rapids are not only natural routes of communication but also spots where contact with another supernatural sphere is established...these falls and rapids figure prominently in Indian myths.... they are concerned with aboriginal life and thought, with mythological scenes, with origins of certain native groups or with tales of strange monsters and many uncanny happenings.

G. Reichel-Dolmatoff (1975)

...contact with another supernatural sphere...

## Boys repeating stories of the creation of the falls

*Falls of Yayacopi, Río Apaporis, Vaupés*

All youths learn from older men or directly from the payés the stories concerning the creation of the many great falls and rapids in the rivers of the Colombian Amazonia. Each falls has its own creation myth. Whilst portaging around rapids, frequently an older boy will recite to younger companions what he has learned from his elders. It may be a short story or may take several hours, thus providing a welcome rest period from an arduous day or even days of paddling. In this way also the beliefs of the origins of their surroundings are kept alive.

All rivers are imagined as snakes, their undulating, glistening bodies stretching over the land, their tail ends lying in remote and isolated regions, while their powerful bodies develop into fierce heads at the river mouth. The ripples on the skins of these winding snakes are the falls and rapids...

G. Reichel-Dolmatoff (1975)

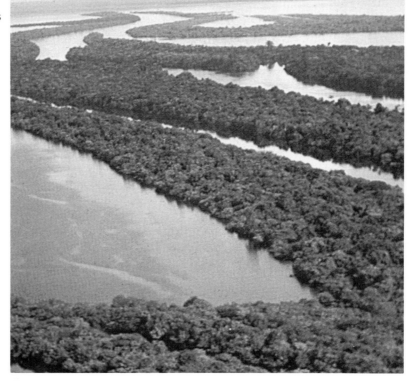

All rivers are imagined as snakes…

## Sinuous branch of the uppermost Río Amazonas

*Leticia, Amazonas*

It is not difficult to understand the Indians' belief in the symbolism of the river, with its constant windings and twistings, as a snake. The symbolism, however, goes much farther and entails the huge anaconda, a water boa, as an important element in creation myths. It was the anaconda who brought the first people from the Milky Way in a canoe. The Tukanoans, for example, recognize two "kinds" of snakes, the land boas and most brightly coloured snakes that may be poisonous; these are interpreted as male elements. The second "kinds" are anacondas and water snakes; these are female elements. As a consequence, rivers are female elements in their mythology.

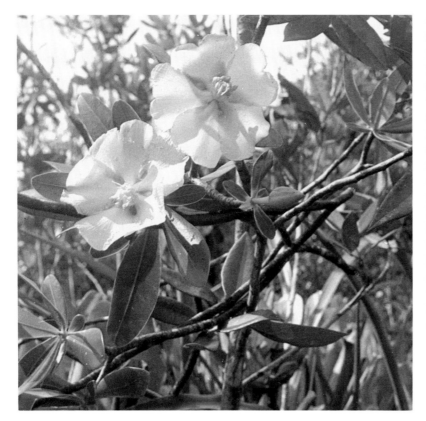

Once, when clambering among the rocks...I came upon a single white flower...which was new to me...the image of that perfect flower remained as persistently in my mind that...I went again in the hope of seeing it still untouched by decay. There was no change...Next day I went again... and after that I went often...and still no faintest sign of change...Why... does not this mystic forest flower fade and perish like the others? I heard from some Indians...that the flower...was called *hata*...they said that it bloomed for the space of moon... And they said that whoso-ever discovered the hata flower... would overcome all enemies and obtain all his desires and finally outlive other men by many years.

W.H. Hudson (1936)

...it blooms for the space of a moon...

## An endemic plant of the ancient sandstone mountains

*Cerro Isibukuri, Río Kananarí, Vaupés*

The many endemic plants found on the numerous sandstone mountains of the Colombian Amazonia have curious uses or are the source of interesting beliefs in their mythological origin. The payés especially enjoy telling their knowledge concerning these plants which, because they are rare or very local, have naturally attracted the Indians' attention.

One such plant is called *ma-né-pa-ree-nee* by the Taiwanos (*Bonnetia holostylis* of the Theaceae or Tea Family) who boil the beautiful flowers in water which is drunk to calm long-standing "pains in the chest". They make special trips to the top of Cerro Isibukuri to gather these flowers which are dried and kept for use when needed.

The Sun Father was "measuring the centre of the day". The equator is...a zone of verticality (when one stands on the equator and notices that all constellations appear to rise and set vertically) and this is why the Creator chose this place. The momentous act of the Sun Father's visit was commemorated...by bygone generations...who carved a number of petroglyphs.... The Rock of *Nyi* is adorned with some of the best-preserved petroglyphs in the entire Vaupés area.... The design shows a triangular face...at the foot of the rock are several other designs...said to be the imprints of the Sun Father's blow gun or the flutes he carried with him.

G. Reichel-Dolmatoff (1975)

...the imprints of the Sun Father's blowgun...

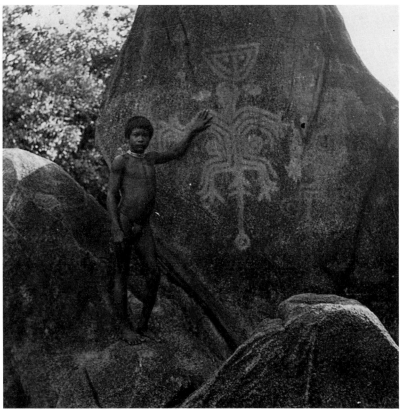

# *Nyi*, god of the rivers

*Río Piraparaná, Vaupés*

This beautiful rock engraving is undoubtedly the most elaborate petroglyph in the Colombian Amazonia. It is sacred to all of the Indians of a wide area. Located near the confluence of the Río Piraparaná with the Apaporis, it is almost on the equator. Carved in hard granite in the remote past, the Indians of today believe that it marks the exact spot where the "first people" came from the Milky Way in a dugout canoe drawn by an anaconda snake—a man, a woman, and three plants: yuca, coca and yajé or caapi.

How ancient this petroglyph is or which Indians made it are unknown. The difficulties of engraving this design on hard granite without modern tools and in a locality which, in high water, is a rapids make even more striking this real work of native art. There is no wonder why it is considered sacred.

# *Euterpe oleracea*, source of edible fruit

*Río Guainía, Vaupés*

The many Indians of the northwest Amazon have a rather vague religion with no gods in the usual sense but a host of anthropomorphic spirits, many being supernatural ancestor beings. The plants most frequently associated with the attempts on the part of the payés or the ordinary Indians to deal with these supernatural forces are the hallucinogens. There are, however, many plants with no psychoactivity that enter into magico-religious symbolism or ritual and which are considered to be directly or indirectly connected with the powers that rule human affairs. Some of them are palms.

The Indians of the Río Guainía who harvest *piassaba* or *chiquichique* fibre (Leopoldinia) believe that an evil spirit, the Kurupira, inhabits the piassaba groves by night in the form of snakes. For this reason, they always work in the groves by day in groups.

Although the leaves of the diminutive Lepidocaryum are best for thatching, substitute materials are often used, because the payés must go through elaborate rituals apparently to protect the boys who collect them from this evil spirit, usually a huge monster, who can assume the form of a palm.

Witoto payés believe that the long spines on the trunk of Astrocaryum are the most potent invisible darts shot into human beings to cause sickness. Before treating the patient, the payé drinks a beverage made from *mirití* (Mauritia) which is believed to enable him to counteract this evil hex.

The Yukunas believe that this mirití represents a spirit that came with the "first people", a dwarf who taught the art of weaving.

The Kai-ya-ree Dance of the Yukunas is held at the time of harvest of the *chontaduro* palm (Guilielma).

The Taiwano payés recommend the trunks of the *cajuayá* (Mauritiella) for house posts, since this palm always waves in the wind and points to the supernatural realm.

These and many similar beliefs indicate that the Indians accord palms a very special place in their mythology and superstition.

...no family of trees is more similar; generically and specifically, none is more varied, even though other families include a greater number of species.

Prof. and Mrs. L. Agassiz (1868)

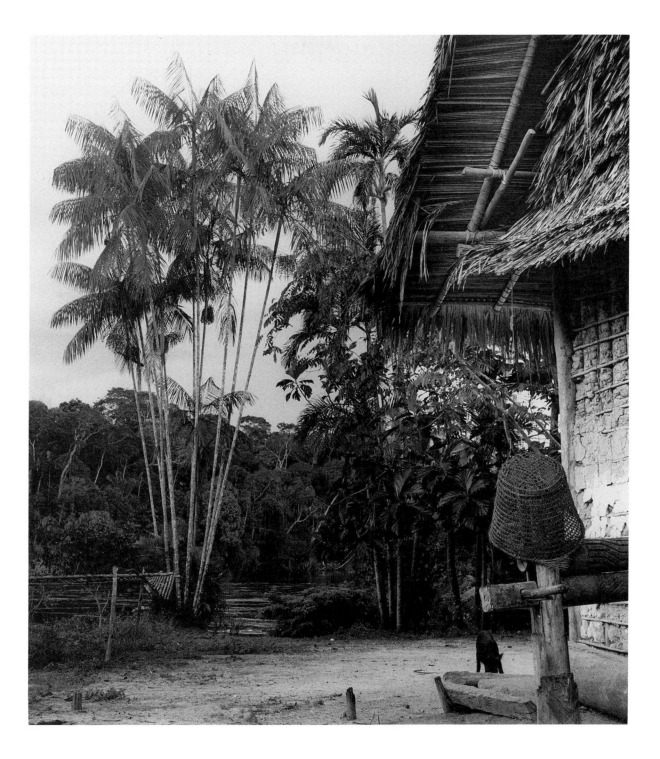

no family…is more similar,…none is…specifically more varied….

The term demon should be applied only to a spirit that may be defined as an individualized supernatural being that is unique of its kind or is strictly localised...

A. Métraux (1949)

# A small palm inhabited by tiny demons

*Cerro Circasia, Río Vaupés, Vaupés*

This small palm is an endemic species and genus (*Parascheelia anchistropetala*), known only from the sandy caatingas at the base of the Cerro Circasia on the Río Vaupés. The woody spathe is located at the very base of the leaves which are only six to ten feet long and which grow out of the soil. Palms attract the attention of the Indians, and the unusual sessile habit of this species has given rise to the firm belief that "little men" live in the spathe. No Indian will camp in the open sandy area where this palm grows for fear of being bewitched or even killed during sleep by these tiny demons.

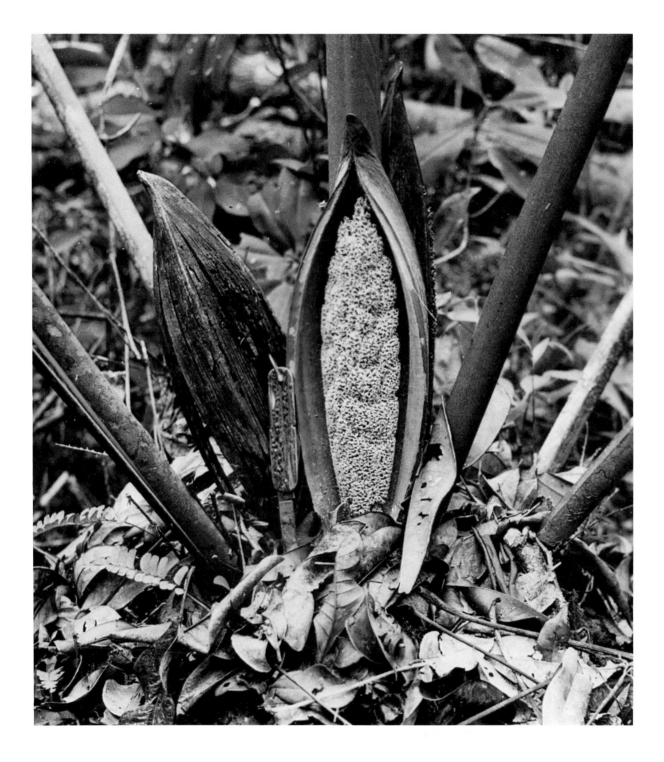

...a supernatural being that...is strictly localized...

Of some payés it is said that they can turn into anacondas which then take on the appearance of large manioc squeezers, the elongated sleeve-like instruments the Indians use to press out the poisonous juice of the grated manioc. The parallel is obvious: The elastic basketry press is compared to the strangling coils of the huge snake. These supernatural manioc squeezers are said sometimes to float in the river, turn into anacondas and devour their victims.

G. Reichel-Dolmatoff (1975)

# Manioc squeezers and anaconda snakes

*Río Kuduyarí, Vaupés*

One of the most curious beliefs propagated by the payés holds that the manioc squeezer (known as the *tipitipi*), a basic invention for pressing the toxic cyanoglycoside from the poisonous yuca, can turn into an anaconda and devour its victims. This transformation can take place at the behest of a payé. Many Indians do not believe this story, but the belief and its many ramifications are constantly discussed in gatherings of the Indians.

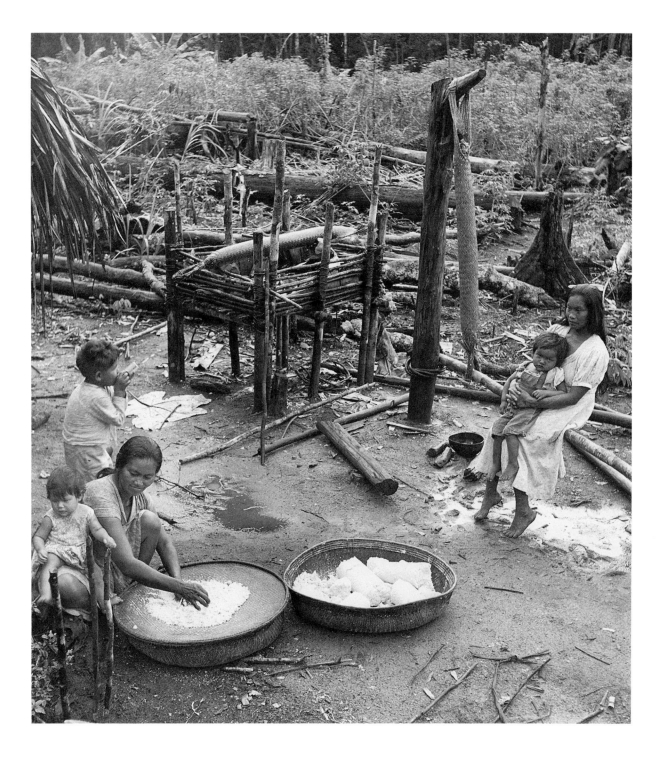

...these manioc squeezers...turn into anacondas...

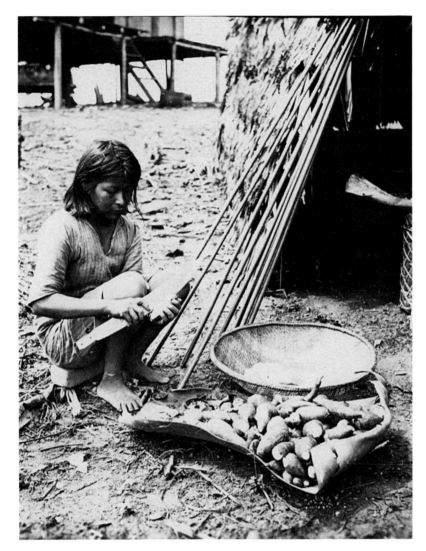

The women recognise the various kinds of *yuca* (*Manihot*) by the colour of the petiole, bark and tuber and by their different mythological origins. Some of the names of these kinds refer to the colour and origins and are very important in ritual dances and in the diet of the shaman when he is about to begin his usual curing seances.

C. LaRotta (1983)

...important in ritual dances and...the diet of the shaman...

# The various "kinds" of yuca

*General in the Colombian Amazonia*

As the principal carbohydrate source of Amazonian diets, yuca has naturally acquired a folklore all its own. It has been a cultigen so long that it is unknown in the wild state and has developed a large number of local ecotypes which the Indians can readily identify, primarily by colour variations. These sundry ecotypes or strains have often very specific names in dances, shamanism and the tales of origin of this most important food plant.

The witch doctors of the Kubeo Indians attach magical significance to the red colouring matter in the spathe of this species (*Philodendron haematinum*). They dye their hands red by handling the spathes before treating a patient.

T. Plowman (1969)

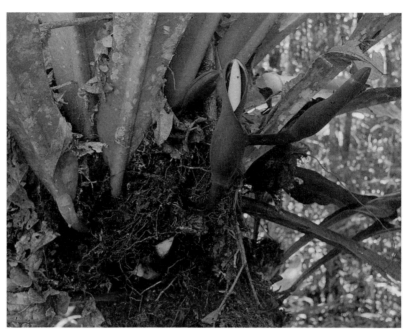

…magical significance to the red colouring matter…

# Red, a magic colour

*Throughout the Colombian Amazonia*

Red seems to have acquired in the Indian mind a very important place. This may be due to the belief that it is somehow significant, since blood is regarded as representing animal and human life. Medicine men anoint their hands with the red dye present in this epiphytic Philodendron of the Araceae or the Aroid Family. The Kubeos chew the raw stem of *Schiekia orinocensis* of the Haemodoraceae or Bloodwort Family to treat bleeding gums and drink a tea of the root to correct "poor blood". Numerous tribes paint new-born babies with red designs made with dye from the achiote plant, *Bixa Orellana* of the Bixaceae or Achiote Family. The purpose of this painting is to ensure healthy growth and freedom from hexing. There are other superstitious uses of plants with reddish or deep orange flowers, stems, roots or latex, their use connected with bleeding or the healing of wounds, suggestive of possible association of the colour with blood.

The brilliant red pigment in *Philodendron haematinum* is due to pelargonidin a precursor of anthocyanins, widespread in the family.

It was never clear to me whether the love charm *pedidya*, a blossom worn in the hair, was intended to work by magic or merely by suggestion. The most effective love potions...are secret and magical.

I. Goldman (1963)

# A magical plant of the savannah

*Falls of Jerijerimo, Río Apaporis, Vaupés*

The resin of either *Retiniphyllum concolor* or *R. truncatum* (Rubiaceae) is an important medicinal of the Taiwanos for treating hemorrhoids and rectal bleeding. The resin must be taken from the fresh plant. Medicine men of the Makuna tribe employ it in magical rites. Amongst the Kubeos, the flowers, worn in the hair, are a potent love charm.

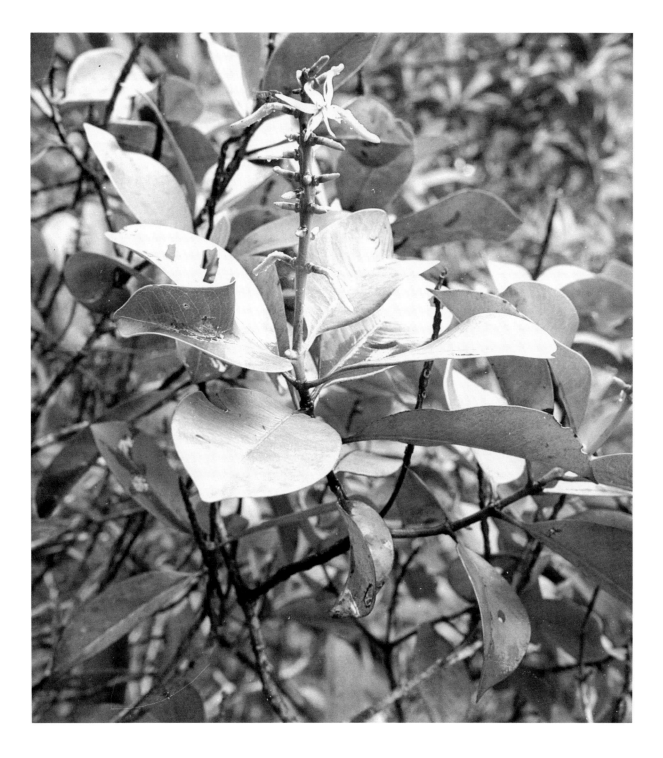

...love potions...are secret and magical.

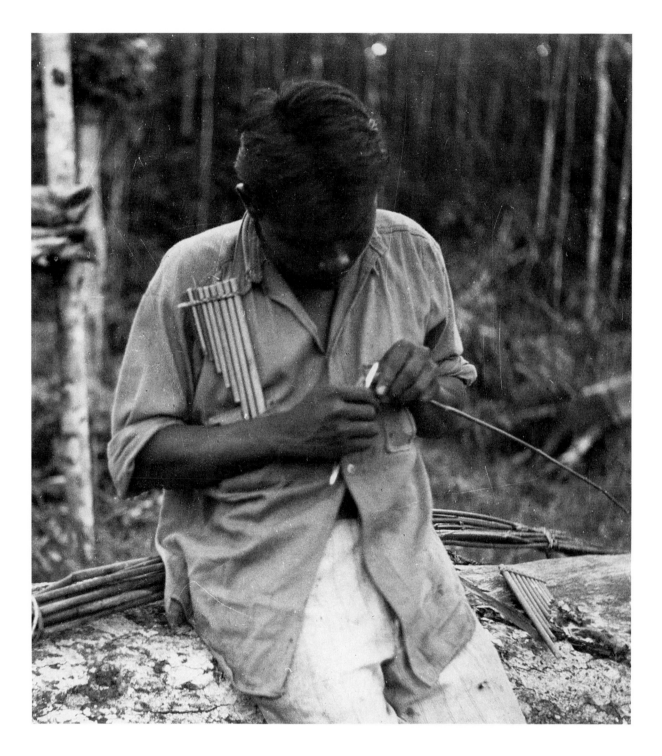

...music...with wind instruments...

Most music is made with wind
instruments: panpipes with three
to thirteen tubes...

J.H. Steward and
A. Métraux (1948)

## Taiwano making a set of panpipes

*Río Kananarí, Vaupés*

Panpipes are an essential part of the music for dances. The
monotonous pentatonic but melodic music, played usually by
youths, helps to keep the dancers in rhythmic unity, but frequently it may be called upon by the shaman to accompany his
chanting, especially when he sings the mythological history of the
creation of the world and the origin of his people.

At night, the young boys play
their pipes...and the clear notes
carry across the still forest.

B. Moser and D. Tayler (1965)

# Makuna panpipe players

*Río Piraparaná, Vaupés*

Panpipe music for the ceremonial dances is almost always provided by boys who usually learn to play the instrument at an early
age. They often get together in the round house of an evening to
practise or to enjoy playing. When they provide music for the
dances, it is invariably the payé who, in a long chanted recital,
expresses his appreciation to the musicians. He explains the
mythological origins of the panpipes and tells the group that the
sounds that they make are pleasant to the supernatural realms to
which the music ascends during the magico-religious rituals
presided over by the payé.

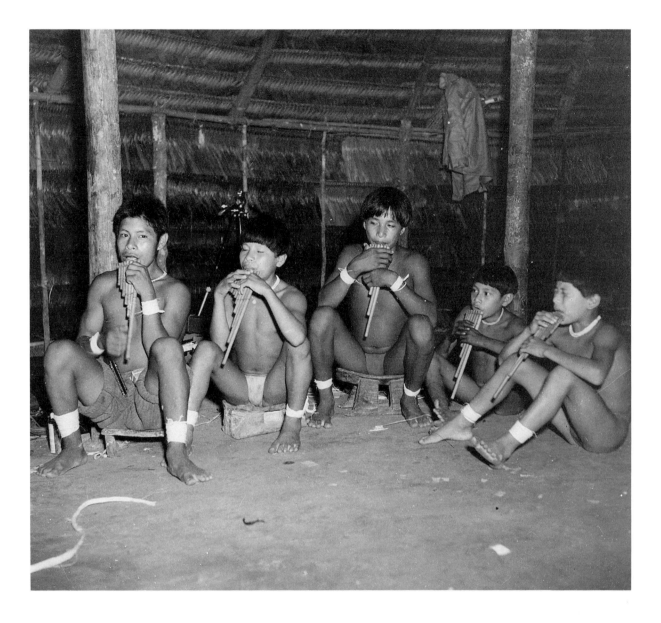

clear notes…across the still forest.

"What good do you think my remedies would be if I didn't sing to them?" The Indians who taught me their secrets believed that words carried by the breath of their shaman have creative power all their own.

F.B. Lamb (1985)

# Tukano singing to three kinds of caapi

*Río Vaupés, Vaupés*

Music is necessary in shamanistic activity throughout the northwest Amazonia. Chants of the payés and panpipes played before and during magico-religious ceremonies are essential. Many of the chants and musical offertories are directed to sacred hallucinogenic plants, Virola and Banisteriopsis, sources of psychoactive snuff and an intoxicating beverage, caapi, respectively. The natives insist that the plants, or the spirits residing within the plants, are pleased with the musical attention.

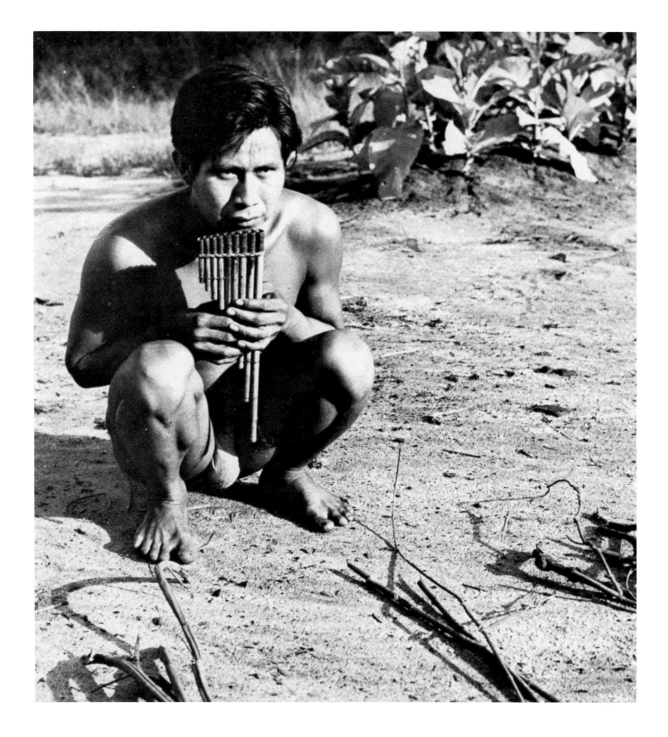

…words…of their shaman have creative power…

The leg rattles are made of polished nutshells.... The nutshells vary in size and shape, though all are approximately bell-like when cut and strung on fibre threads. They give a tinkling sound if shaken....

T. Whiffen (1915)

# Source of leg rattles

*Jinogojé, Río Apaporis, Vaupés*

In various parts of the Colombian Amazonia, several different plants with hard-shelled fruits are employed in making leg rattles for dancing. In the Vaupés, the favourite plant is a member of the Gourd Family which is cultivated, usually near the houses and frequently, it is said, under the watchful eye of the local medicine man. The rattles are tied to the lower part of the leg; together with hand rattles, panpipes and sometimes hollow thumping sticks, they provide a not unpleasant tinkling accompaniment.

The plant which is pictured represents a species new to botanical science; it was described and given its technical name—*Cayaponia kathematophora*—a species epithet from the Greek term meaning "music bearing".

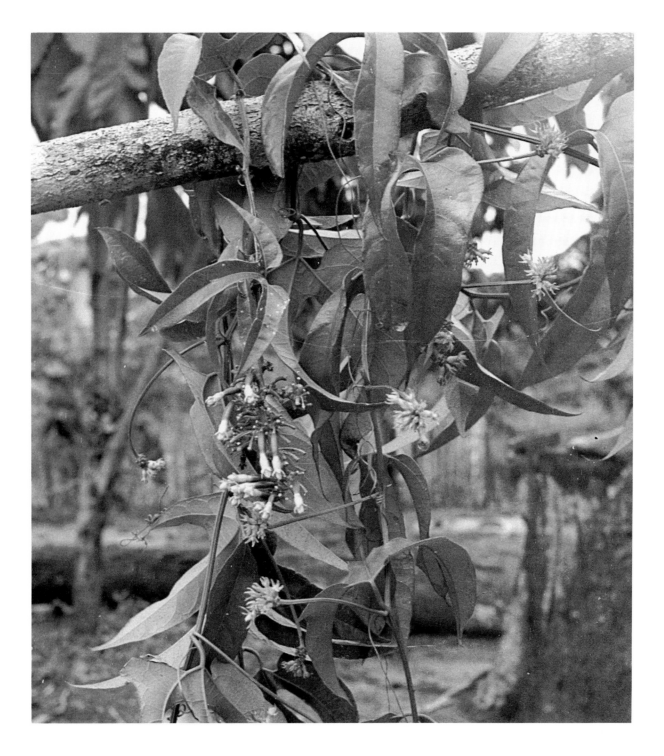

...a tinkling sound if shaken....

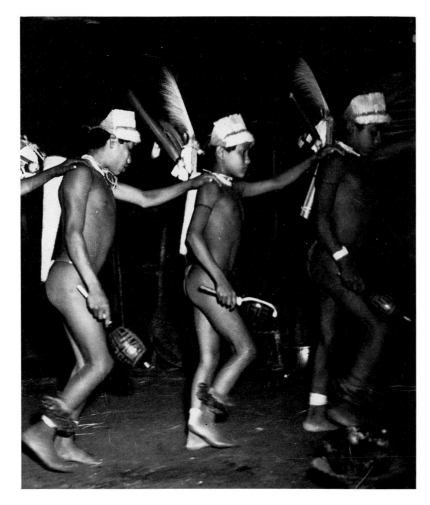

In their right hands all participants held a gourd rattle decorated with designs scratched on the surface and decorated with feathers which, in addition to anklet rattles, served to accompany the stamping of the right foot and thereby emphasize even more the strong rhythm of the dance.

T. Koch-Grünberg (1909)

...the strong rhythm of the dance.

## Makuna boys with rattles

*Río Piraparaná, Vaupés*

The Indian usually has a strong sense of rhythm. At an early age, boys begin to learn to use various instruments to provide cadence and beauty to the dance. Hand rattles are extremely important, since they serve also as one of the tools often employed by the shaman to accompany his chanting and invocations to counteract or expel the malevolent spirit that has caused sickness. The designs frequently painted on the gourd of the rattle, sometimes copies of the figures found on rock engraving in the rivers, are considered to represent sacred symbols and are usually executed after consultation with a payé.

172

Most famous of all the dances is the *Yurupari*, a ceremony performed only by men.

P.H. Allen (1947)

...a ceremony performed only by men.

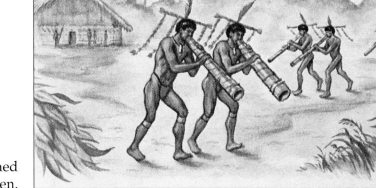

# Yuruparí Dance amongst the Kubeos

*Río Vaupés, Vaupés*

The term *yuruparí* has been employed in the literature in many ways and has been translated as representing "the devil", "ancestor spirit", "mystery", "fertility rite", "initiation ritual", "creation god", "harvest insurance" and other supernatural concepts. Yuruparí Dances are widespread, especially in the western Amazonia and upper Orínoquia. They all characteristically use sacred bark horns and are taboo to women.

Women are forbidden to see them and, at the first sound of the instruments, all flee to the forests; in former times, women who did accidentally see a horn were killed, usually with poison. The horns are hidden between the dances, oftentimes in the sandy bottoms of brooks from which the payés remove them when needed. The older men open boxes of feather ornaments to decorate the horns whilst they are in use. The youngest initiants must undergo severe whippings by the payés and masters of the dance, usually drawing blood; they are shown where the trumpets are hidden and, with this ritual, are separated from boyhood and become men. The dance steps are led by the payés who frequently pass around a two-foot long cigar for all to smoke and who lead in the chanting which mingles with the explosive sounds of the sacred horns.

...the most important and dramatic dances are not the more or less open and profane ones, without masks, but the more private, secret and sacred, masked dances.... There were dances depicting the butterfly... the buzzard, the jaguar, various fishes, larvae, alternating with those depicting evil demons who have taken on human shape or representations of giants or dwarfs.

P. Radin (1942)

# Yukuna Kai-ya-ree dancer with staff rattle

*Río Miritiparaná, Amazonas*

The Kai-ya-ree Dance of the Yukunas and Tanimukas performed during the first week in April of each year could be called a dance of evolution. The four-day series of dances begins with a masked dance depicting the spirit of darkness and propitiating it. This is followed by a long set of dances, each with a special uniform representing numerous animals (butterflies, ants, anteaters, jaguars, fishes, etc.), and ends with a dance in honour of the sun in which circular balsa-wood masks with the face of the sun painted in yellow are worn. Each dance has its own music and songs. A tremendous amount of work goes into the preparation for this long ceremony which is attended by all Indians living within a reasonable distance.

In many ways, the ceremony depicts what we might interpret as the Indians' ideas of evolutionary development of the animal and human races and their conflict with the forces of darkness and their dependence on the forces of light.

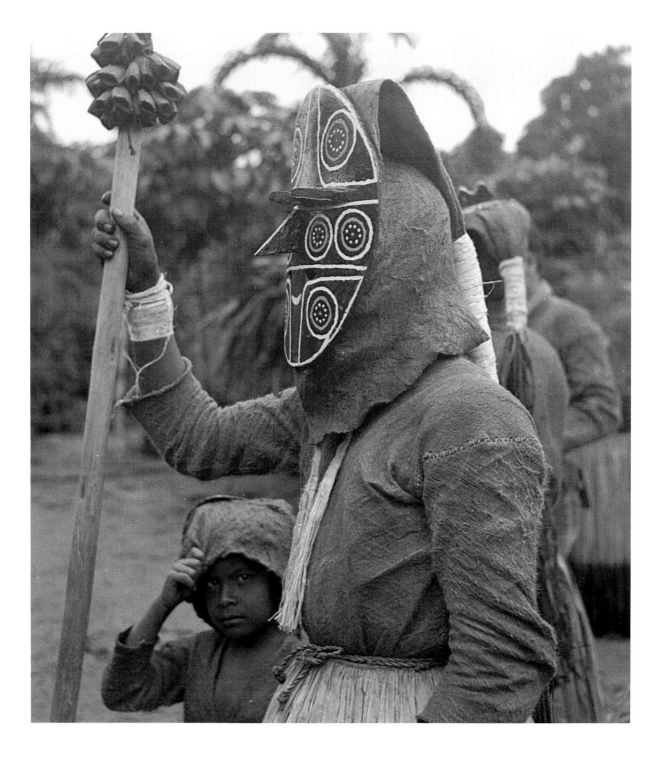

...the most important and dramatic dances are...sacred, masked dances....

The *tunday* or manguaré, the remarkable instrument for signalling or communicating by sound through the forest, is used by various tribes in the Amazon Valley.

W.E. Hardenburg (1912)

# Witotos signalling for a tribal ceremony

*La Chorrera, Río Igaraparaná, Amazonas*

One of the most ingenious objects of the Indians of numerous tribes in the Colombian Amazon is the manguaré or tunday, a signal drum made from a hollowed-out log. One or two trunks of hard wood are hollowed out by burning or charring the interior with very hot stones inserted through a longitudinal slit in the log. If there are two logs, one is referred to as male, the other as female. When the interior is fully charred, the shell varies in thickness from half an inch to five or six inches. This enables the Indian with his rubber-tipped stout drumstick to beat at different points on the outside of the log to obtain different notes.

The manguaré is basically a signal drum, but it may carry many messages: invitations to dances, the place, the purpose of the dance. It has aptly been called the "telegraph drum"; not infrequently, it may be utilized as a musical instrument at dances together with panpipes and rattles.

The thumping sounds can be heard 10 or 12 miles away, sometimes even farther if the sound travels along a river and not through the forest. If other malocas have manguarés, conversations can be carried on. The log or logs are suspended from the rafters or from frames built for the purpose, usually inside the malocas. They are often decorated.

The origin of the manguaré is lost in antiquity. The Indians all say that it was given to them by the "ancient ones"; many are of great age, handed down from one generation to the next.

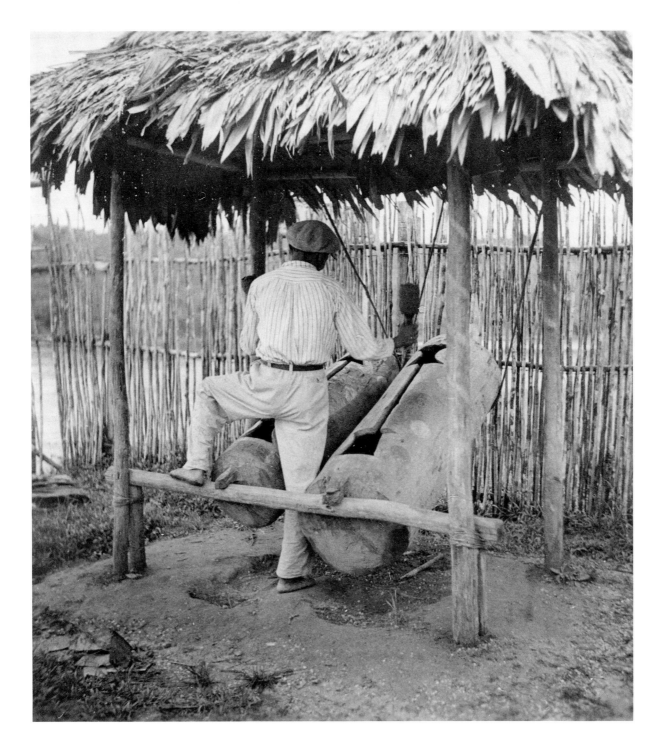

...by sound through the forest...

The demon resides in the mask,
is embodied in it; for the Indian,
the mask is the demon.

T. Koch-Grünberg (1910)

# The Yukuna devil mask

*Río Miritiparaná, Amazonas*

According to Yukuna legend, the first born child of the tribe was conceived by an anaconda who saw the woman eat the seed of the *ye-cha* tree (*Micrandra Spruceana* of the Euphorbiaceae) which looks like an anaconda egg. She became pregnant and eventually bore a boy-child. The woman's brothers, loath to kill the infant, spared him, and he grew up happily and full of glee. But while he was a child by day, he changed into a boa at night.

The first dance in the Kai-ya-ree uses a staff symbolic of trees; the following dances employ a variety of masks representing a great number of animals, from the lowest to the advanced. The Kai-ya-ree is basically a religious ceremony expressing the Indian's beliefs of the origin and evolution of life. These ideas are intricately connected with the interplay of forces of good and evil, for all life is eventually, in his understanding of cosmology, controlled by good and bad demons.

178

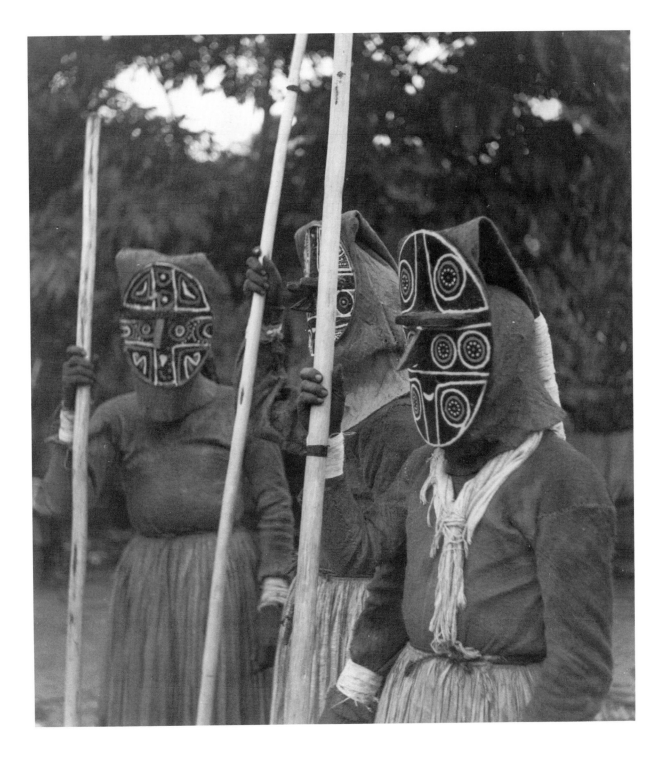

...the mask is the demon.

[They] wear their masks representing the spirits of various animals and plants in an attempt to influence supernatural beings. The rites involve a clearly sexual component illustrated in the text of the songs and the appearance of a dancer with an outsize phallus made of wood, and their function is to stimulate the fertility of the flora and fauna

F. Trupp (1981)

# One of the four-day series of Kai-ya-ree Dances

*Caño Guacayá, Río Miritiparaná, Amazonas*

One of the dances in the long series during the Kai-ya-ree has to do with *Wagti*, one of the spirits, according to the Yukunas, who can be either benevolent or malevolent. This specific dance has sexual overtones, since it celebrates the placating of Wagti for continuing tribal fertility and future success of the crops. The sexual character of the dance is clearly evident as the performers carry wooden representations of the penis.

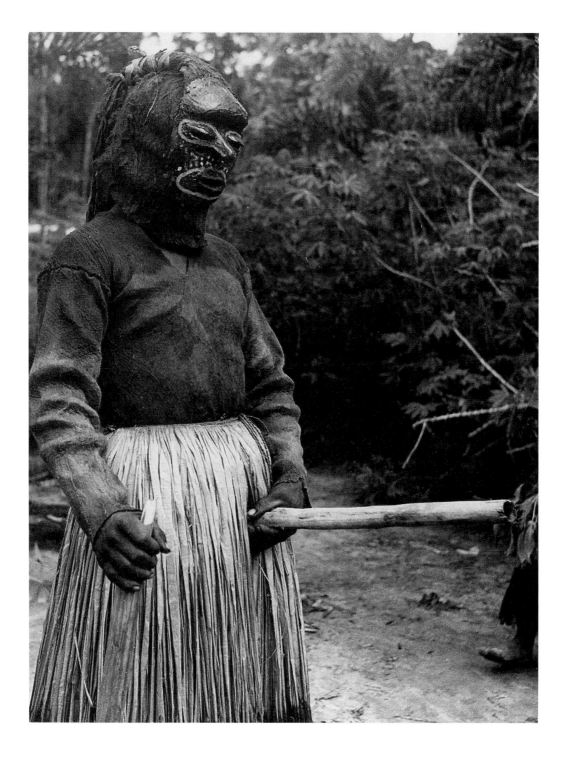

…to stimulate…fertility of the flora and fauna.

Wagti, the devil, was in no sense
the eternal enemy of mankind.
It was Wagti who caused all the
trees and plants of the jungle
to grow. He was the mysterious
creator and vivifier. His moods
were, indeed, changeable.
He could be irate as well as
benevolent, but in no sense was
he the enemy of *Wako*, the "good
god". He was merely the dark
and fearful spirit of the earth.

W.M. McGovern (1927)

# The energetic dance honouring Wagti

*Río Miritiparaná, Amazonas*

The Kai-ya-ree Dance is attended by 80 to 100 Indians who come
from great distances and is held at the time of the harvest of the
peach palm or *chontaduro* fruit (*Guilielma speciosa*) in early April.
The dances last four or even five days, as long as the food and
fermented chicha last. The first in the series of many masked
dances, and one that is repeated several times during the celebration, requires great expenditure of energy because of the many
really beautiful steps that are interspersed with rhythmic stamping; it honors the supernatural creator.

During the Kai-ya-ree, several large dugout canoes are filled with
chicha made, usually, from the starch-rich chontaduro fruits. The
meal or fariña, the carbohydrate staff of life, ordinarily made from
manioc, may also for this festival be made from the chontaduro
fruits or from the seeds of ye-cha (*Micrandra Spruceana*) after their
toxic cyanogenic glycosides have been leached out. Quantities of
smoked game and fish are supplied to all visitors, having been
hunted or fished by the men of the maloca where the celebration
is held and smoked by the women of the house. The entire
intricate preparation is supervised by the payés, since the dance
is considered a sacred ceremony.

182

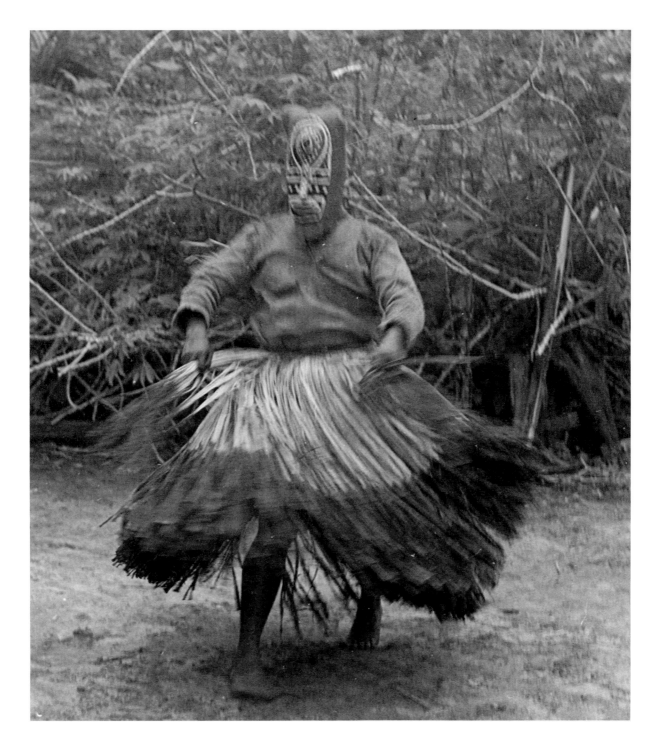

…the dark and fearful spirit of earth.

Tree latex is used...for making torches [and] in the manufacturing of dancing masks.

J.C.T. Uphof (1968)

# The principal source of latex for masks

*Río Apaporis, Vaupés*

The many complicated dancing masks, especially those prepared for the four-day Kai-ya-ree Dance of the Yukunas, are fashioned with care from the resins of various plants. The best of such resins, according to the Yukunas, is that from several species of the genus Moronobea of the Guttiferae or St. John's Wort Family. Other plants with resins used for the same purpose are species of Clusia and Symphonia of this family.

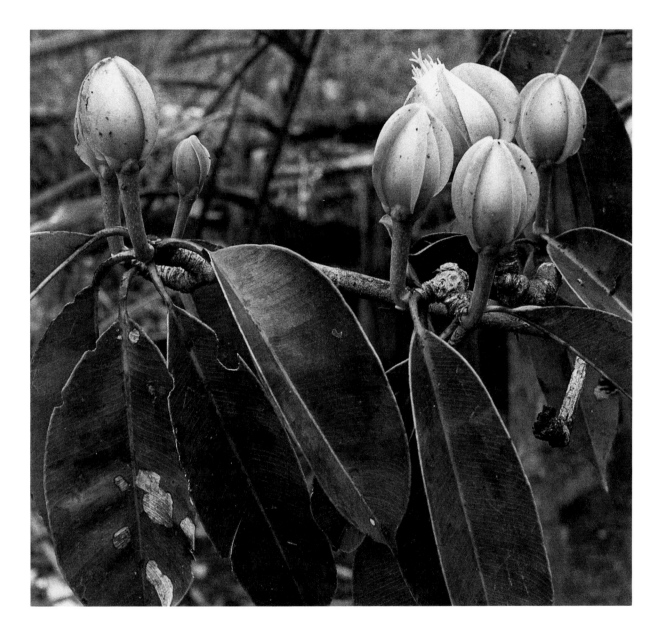

...latex...[for] dancing masks...

[An Indian]...uses his machete to apply the heated resin to the bark-cloth hood and models the actual face of the mask.

F. Trupp (1981)

## Yukuna craftsman preparing Kai-ya-ree mask

*Río Miritiparaná, Amazonas*

The artistry involved in making dancing masks from hot resin is intricate and requires long apprenticeship. The latex must be liquid and applied to bark bases whilst it is still extremely hot. This is all done not with small artist's tools but with a long, cumbersome machete. This operation is one of the many examples of the inherent artistic ability of the Amazon Indians.

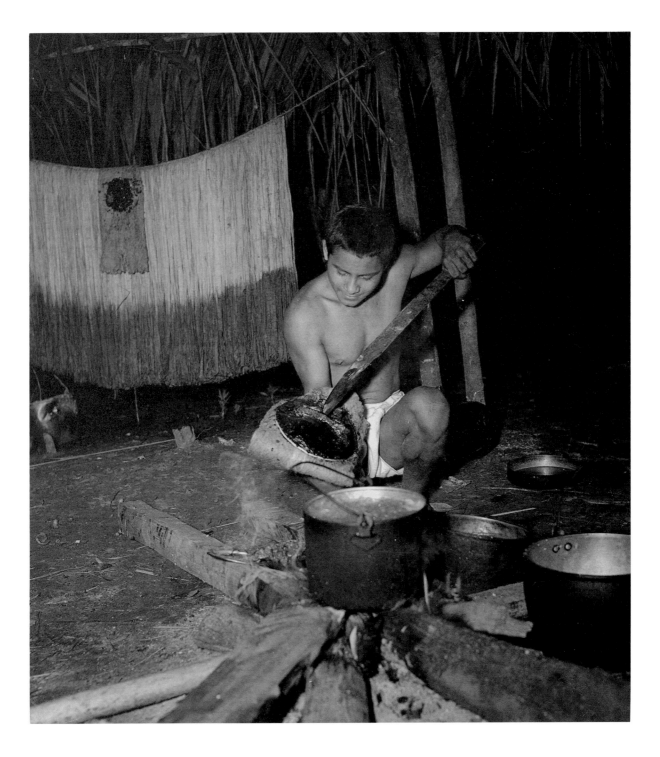

…his machete…[applies] the heated resin to the bark-cloth hood…

To learn more of an Indian's life ...and to visit one of these huts becomes an irresistible desire... the inmate is friendly disposed.... His children are eating the agreeable red and yellow fruits of the peach palm (*Guilielma speciosa*). In the Indian villages, about the houses, many hundreds of trees may often be seen, adding to the beauty of the landscape and supplying an abundance of wholesome food.

B. Seemann (1856)

# Peach palms around an Indian house

*Río Kuduyarí, Vaupés*

The peach palm or chontaduro (*Guilielma speciosa*, sometimes called *Bactris Gasipaes*) is, next to the manioc or tapioca plant, the most important food of the Indians of the northwest Amazon. This palm is an ornamental tree as well as an important food crop. It is planted usually in circular or rectangular rows around the malocas. The extremely nutritious fruit which ripens in late March or early April is an excellent source of carbohydrate and is rich in a tasty oil. It is so important in Amazonian life that it enters into native mythology, and sacred dances are organized at the time of ripening of the fruit.

This cultivated palm is not believed to occur in an undoubted wild state and, while it is presumably native to the westernmost Amazon, its exact place of origin is unknown.

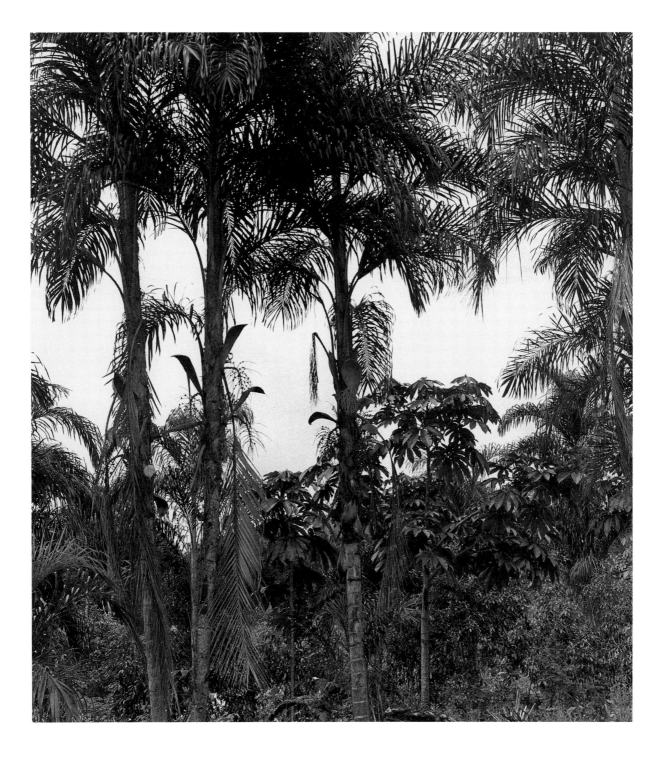

…an abundance of wholesome food.

The deeper meaning of all these masked dances is clear. It is a charm. The spirit of the deceased, to which is everywhere ascribed an angry, revenge-seeking nature, is to be propitiated so that it cannot return and take away one of the bereaved.

T. Koch-Grünberg (1910)

# Uniform for Kubeo Mourning Dance

*Río Kuduyarí, Vaupés*

The garb of the Kubeo Mourning Dance is very different from the uniforms worn in dances for other celebrations. It is more restrictive, and the dances are more subdued. Nevertheless, according to reports, tremendous amounts of chicha are consumed during the funereal celebration; but, since intoxication is considered a sacred or supernatural condition, the drinking does not represent a search for pleasure but rather what may be called a religious sending of the deceased on his final trip.

The dance is characterised by alimentary and sexual restrictions to be observed prior to the ceremony of burial. The payé invariably supervises the entire death ceremony.

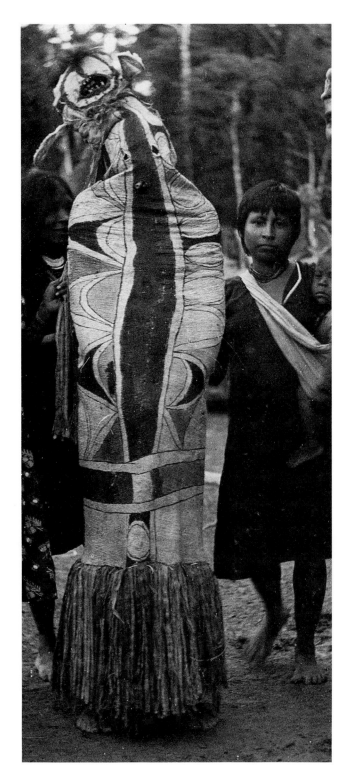

...the spirit of the
deceased...is to be
propitiated...

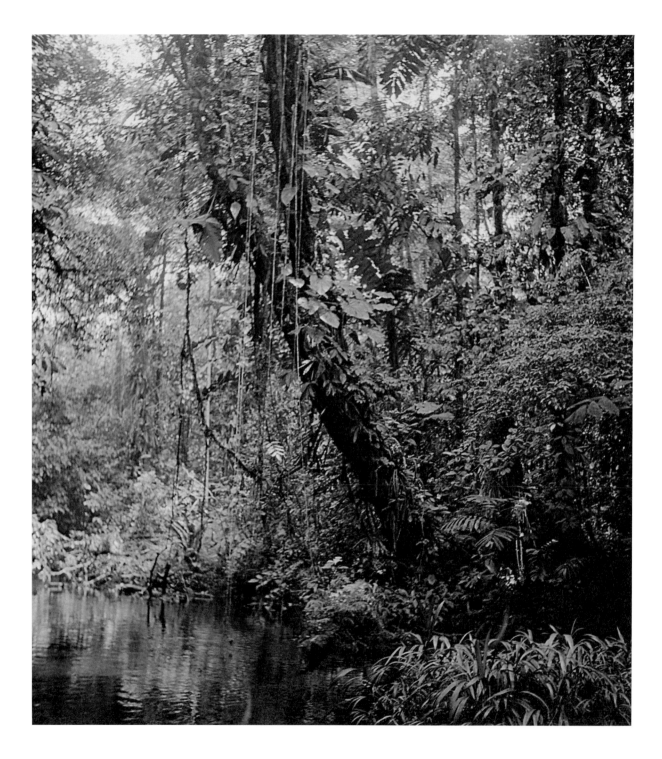

The forest is silent and unchanging…and harbours dangers…

The forest is silent and unchanging. Because of its vast extent it is far less known to the Indian and, therefore, in his mind, harbors more dangers [than the rivers]. As soon as one enters its gloom, one has to adapt oneself to a closer range of things—to the roots and vines, the thorny branches and the slippery trunks that cross stagnant waters.

G. Reichel-Dolmatoff (1975)

## An isolated and suspectful forest locality

*Río Macaya, Vaupés*

Even the botanist who first penetrates the Amazonian forests is amazed by their overwhelming richness, exuberance and novelty. Those native-born and raised in this environment never forget to hold it in reverence and to protect it, even though they believe that supernatural beings frequent certain places in it, awaiting human trespassers to waylay.

In many respects the forest dweller is our most efficient conservationist.

Trees often, and other types
of plants less frequently, are
regarded with reverence or as
sacred for a variety of reasons.
In some cases, the reason is lost
in the antiquity of the people.

J.M. Watt (1972)

# A stilt-rooted tree

*Jinogojé, Río Apaporis, Vaupés*

Many who have not worked with the forest-dwelling Indians of
the Amazon might not understand their fear of certain "beings"
in the jungle. It is, however, true that, together with their respect
for the dense vegetation, there are certain trees and sparse areas
which, for personal safety, they must avoid. For some reason,
which we could not understand, our natives hesitated to fell a tree
with stilt roots, explaining that "it was not like other trees." We
assumed that their hesitancy was due to the fact that, as with other
unusual plants, there was some special importance attached to it
in nature.

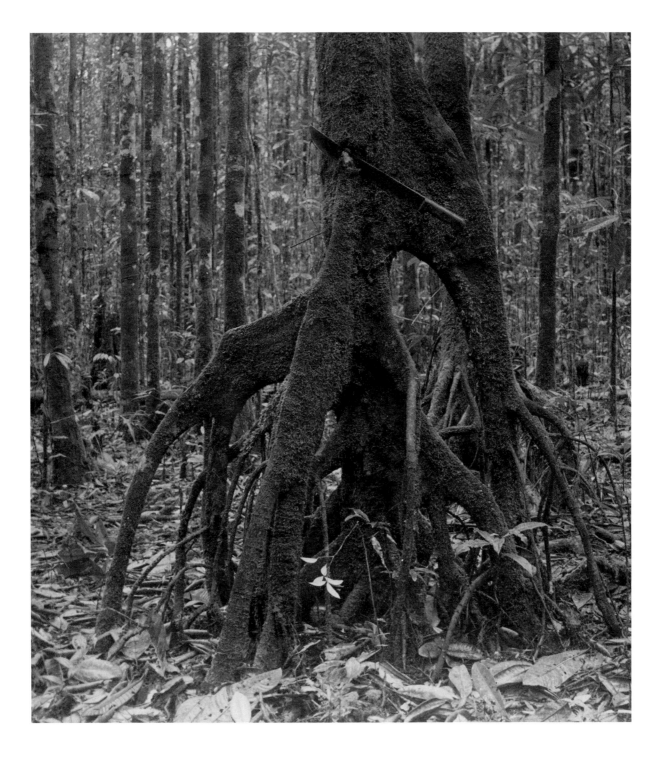

Trees…are regarded with reverence or as sacred…

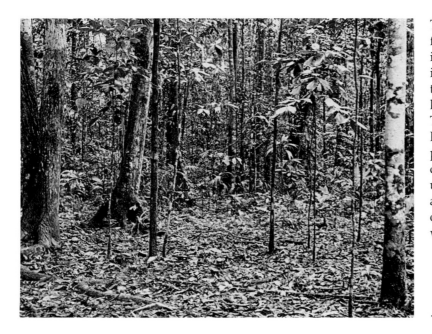

There are...dangerous spots in the forest. Sometimes one finds a clearing, often quite large, where there is hardly any plant growth or where the flat ground is covered by low herbs but lacks trees or underbrush. These spots...are feared by the Indians;...they are the gathering places of spirits, of the souls of the dead or of ghostly apparitions of unknown origin. Uncanny noises are heard there, and should someone come near such a clearing, he will run the danger of falling ill.

G. Reichel-Dolmatoff (1975)

...gathering places of the spirits...

# The "Garden of the Devil"

*Puerto Ospina, Río Putumayo, Putumayo*

One finds clear areas in the dense jungle which are well known to the Indians and their hunters who say they are full of unforeseeable dangers, many of which cannot be avoided in the course of normal activities. Many of these areas are known as "Gardens of the Devil". They are inhabited by ant-infested and toxic shrubs or small trees of the genus Duroia. Nothing else will grow where they thrive, except Selaginella and a few ferns. Such spots certainly look deserted and forlorn.

There has been no scientific explanation of this unusual environmental occurrence. The Indian believes that it has a supernatural cause—the residence of invisible beings.

Some assume that the ferocious ants living in Duroia devastate the plant life that would invade the region around their homes; others explain that Duroia may exude a substance toxic to other vegetation; still others presume that the soil in these isolated spots is different. We are left with the improbable indigenous supposition that their origin is supernatural. It is one of the scientific enigmas of the region.

All these falls and rapids figure prominently in the Indian myths and traditions.... The Jerijerimo Falls...is a most extraordinary sight:...deep in the forests of one of the least known regions of the Vaupés territory.

G. Reichel-Dolmatoff (1975)

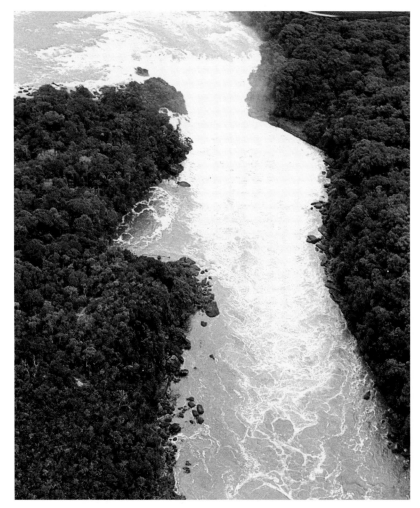

...a most extraordinary sight...

## Jerijerimo Falls

*Río Apaporis, Vaupés*

The Río Apaporis is largely peaceful, yet occasionally it becomes a thunderous river 1350 miles in length. It is interrupted by many beautiful yet dangerous rapids and waterfalls. These are caused by the numerous sandstone mountains in the area and their rocky bases. However, they are explained by the Indians to be of ancient, supernatural origin, raised up by powerful shamans of the past or by spirits who needed boundary markers. Each of the major rapids is sacred to a group of modern Indians. Jerijerimo is sacred to the Taiwanos who live nearby on the Río Kananarí.

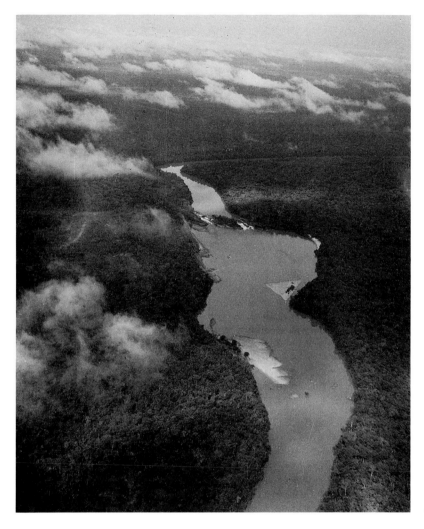

Whereas the forest is undifferentiated terrain, the rivers are known to every turn and outcrop of rock .... The river is the source of the ancestral powers, of benefits as well as of dangers.... The river is literally and symbolically a binding thread for the people. It is a source of emergence and the path along which the ancestors had travelled. It contains in its place names genealogical as well as mythological references, the latter at the petroglyphs in particular.

I. Goldman (1963)

...the path along which the ancestors had travelled.

# The sacred region of Jerijerimo

*Falls of Jerijerimo, Río Apaporis, Vaupés*

The rivers are extremely important in the mythology and superstition of the Indians. They are the homes of innumerable supernatural beings, many of whom must be consulted, appeased and pacified by the shaman's intervention. These spiritual beings are especially active in the vicinity of the numerous rapids of the rivers where, naturally, men are in greater danger than in the placid waters. It is usually the Master of the Fish who must be placated by the payé's pleas, although there are other and lesser spirits operating in the rivers and smaller waterways.

Waterfalls and rapids often function as territorial borders and mythical sites...the Indians regard these...as the birthplaces of the different tribes or as the abode of the "Lord of the Fish."

F. Trupp (1981)

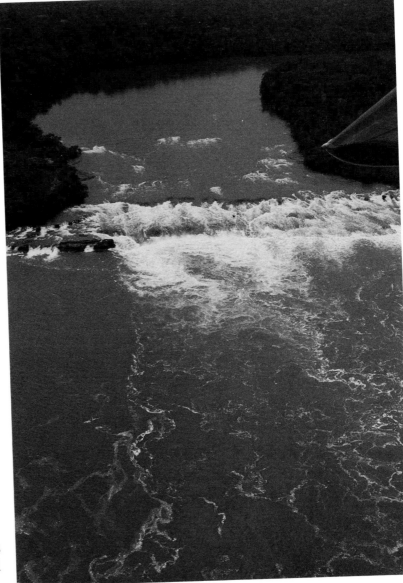

Waterfalls...function as territorial borders and mythical sites.

# Falls of Yuruparí

*Site of the Kubeo Yuruparí Dance*

This beautiful waterfall, the uppermost of the Río Vaupés, is sacred to the Kubeo Indians who annually hold the principal Yuruparí Dance of the year at this location. It is so important in tribal life that Indians often travel days to attend the ceremony.

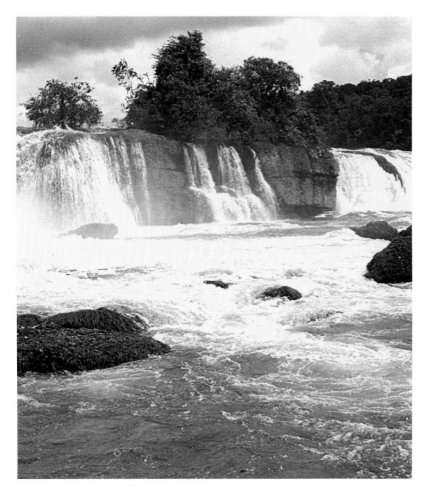

For many of the rapids, rivers, islands, canals, rocks, mountains, forests, etc., the Indians assume a mythical origin.

A. Brüzzi A. da S. (1962)

...a mythical origin.

# Falls of Yayacopi

*Río Apaporis, Vaupés*

The beautiful horseshoe-shaped falls of Yayacopi are sacred to the Makuna Indians of the Ríos Piraparaná and Popeyaká. Together with the Falls of Jerijerimo slightly upstream, they are in a locality of great interest to the naturalist as an area of many endemic plants found nowhere else. The Indians, knowing this, shared their perspicacious observations with the botanists collecting representative plants of this rich flora.

The Makuna origin myths explain how the gods erected this great barrier as a boundary marker for their parcel of a territorial home when they came from the Milky Way to populate the earth.

The legend of the *mai-d'agua* ("Mother of the Waters") is... artless: this faery enchantress frequents rivers and the sombre *igarapés* [channels]. She waylays young couples and brings them bad luck...she sings her magic chants. The Indian who tries to see the Mother of Waters is struck with delirium. Scarcely have his eyes gazed upon her beauty than he is deprived of his senses and thrown into transports of delight ...and if he lets himself be thus drawn away and looks for her on the banks of the river, the faery opens her beautiful arms among the weeds, twines them around him and makes him die of love in the bed of the river.

Baron de Santa-Ana Nery (1901)

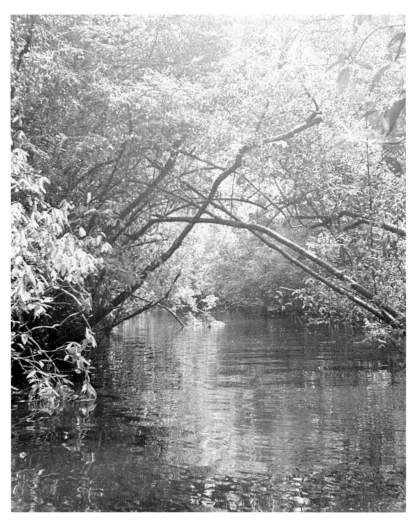

She sings her magic chants.

## Supernatural dangers in the waterways

*San Felipe, Río Negro, Vaupés*

The dark and sluggish canals and creeks, where the vegetation practically takes over, seem to be regions where the Indian believes that dangerous spirits and demons ply their nefarious antics. These locations are wonderful collection sites for botanists. Our native helpers went with us, however, feeling safe because there were three or four individuals in the party and because the botanists were not Indians. But fear of sluggish waterways draped with overhanging vegetation is very strong, especially towards twilight.

The rocky hills one encounters... in the depths of the forest are feared by the Indians who believe that it is there that the supernatural masters of the game animals have their abodes. These hills...are thought to be the malocas wherein the animals live under the protection of their master, and near these hills...are open spots, where they are said to gather to dance and play.

G. Reichel-Dolmatoff (1975)

# One end of Cerro Chiribiquete

*Río Macaya, Vaupés*

The flat quartzitic mountains in the Colombian Amazonia are stark elevations in an otherwise flat tropical forest. The home of an extraordinary number of endemic plants, they are remnants of a once continuous range of elevations stretching in a sort of crescent from the mountains of the Guianas and southern Venezuela to the mountains of La Macarena in Colombia, close to the much younger Andes.

These mountains of strange shapes and different floras have long puzzled the native people, and there can be no wonder why their shamans have decided that they are the homes of supernatural beings.

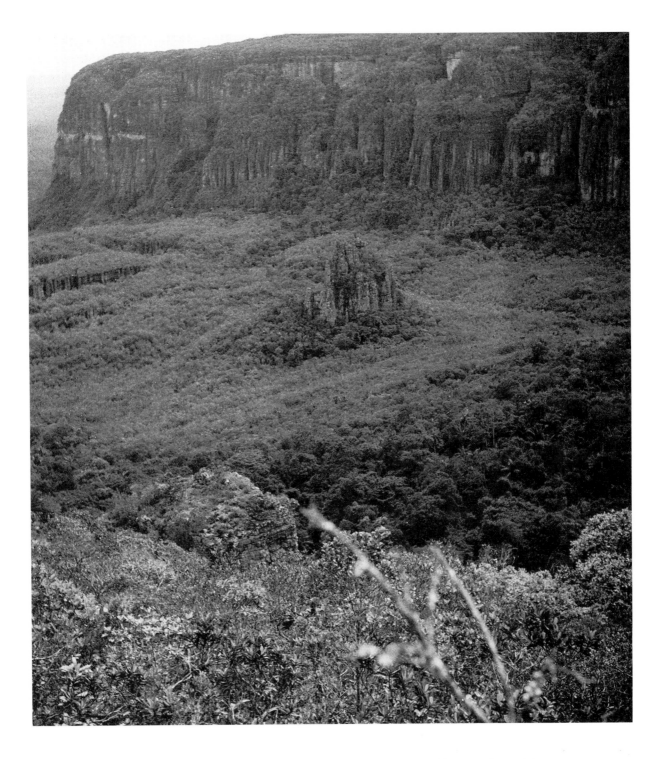

...the rocky hills...are feared by the Indians...

The forests and the rivers, they believe, are populated by a multitude of dangerous spirits — devils or monsters — some of which pursue humans to kill them...the best known spirit and the most feared is the *boráro*... commonly called *kurupira*...but there are other beings that dwell in the forest...[In a] very distinct category are those called *uaxtí*, of which there are two groups — the uaxtí of the forest...and those of the water...both the boráro and the uaxtí are creatures that live in the depths of the jungle.

G. Reichel-Dolmatoff (1968)

# Forests of Chiribiquete and the Río Ajaju

*Confluence of the Ríos Ajaju and Macaya, Vaupés*

River symbolism amongst the Tukanoan Indians is very complex because the imagery refers to different contexts, each with its own code of interpretation. In one image the river is conceived as an elongated tangle of vines, the main stream; and its many branches and oxbows representing the entwined stems of the jungle "vine of the soul".

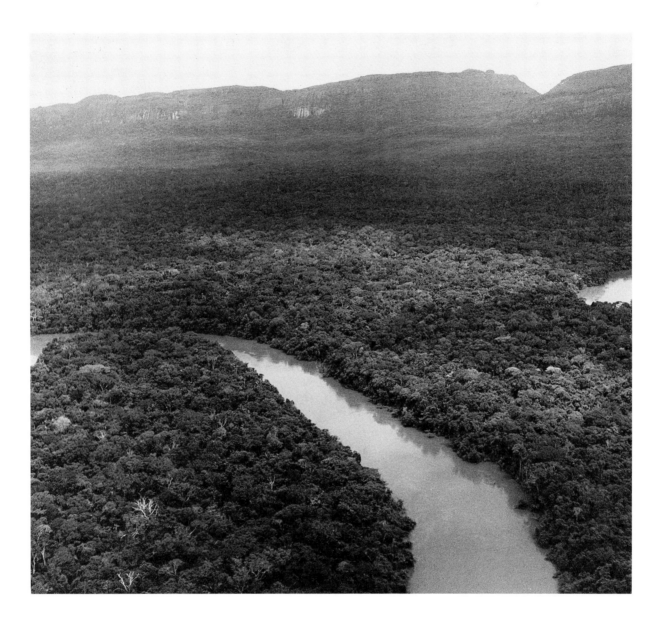

The forests and rivers [have] a multitude of dangerous spirits…

These hills, with their cliffs and
dark recesses, are...the dwelling
places of *Vai-mahsë*, the supernatural Master of Animals..., a
payé in his own right....This spirit
being...is generally imagined and
seen in hallucinations as a red
dwarf, a small person in the attire
of a hunter armed with a bow
and arrow.

G. Reichel-Dolmatoff (1975)

# Tangled mountain vegetation

*Summit of Cerro Isibukuri, Río Kananarí, Vaupés*

The flat summits of the sandstone mountains are clad with a
tangled growth of shrubby plants, many of which are of great
botanical interest as endemic species found nowhere else. The
Indian, accustomed to the high forests through which it is usually
easy to walk, does not enjoy the closed vegetation through which
he cannot see and in which he believes monsters may find it easy
to hide.

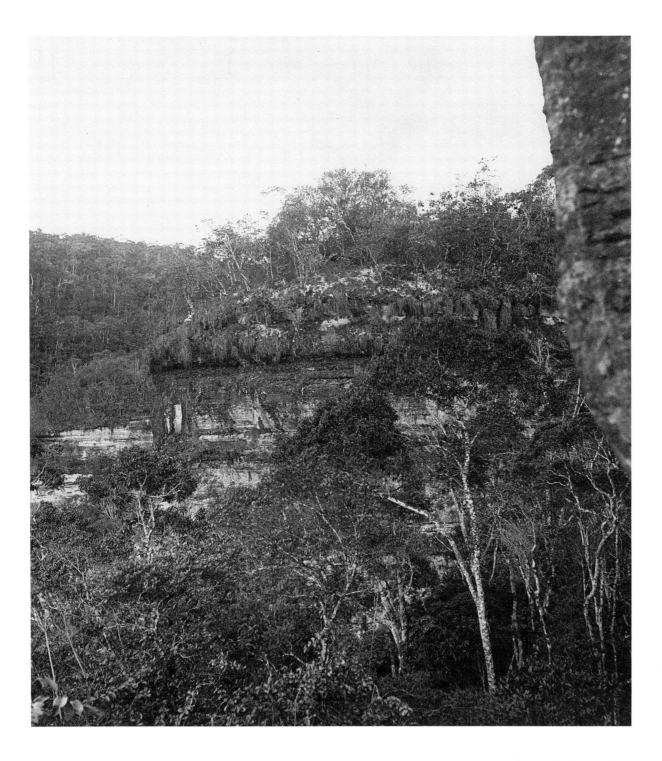

…dwelling places of the Master of Animals…

[The Colombian Amazonia] is characterized by the flat-topped mountains called *mesetas*. These mountains, which are covered with dense vegetation, are remnants of the Guiana Shield and play an important part in the Indian mythology.

F. Trupp (1981)

# The summit of Cerro Isibukuri

*Río Kananarí, Vaupés*

The strange endemic flora on the isolated sandstone mesetas, related to the flora on the *tepuís* of Venezuela and the Guianas, is recognised by the Indians as different from the vegetation of the jungles of the flat country surrounding these mountains. Many tales have grown up around some of the unusual plants of the low, tangled floras of these extraordinary areas, most of them figuring in the rich folklore of mythology.

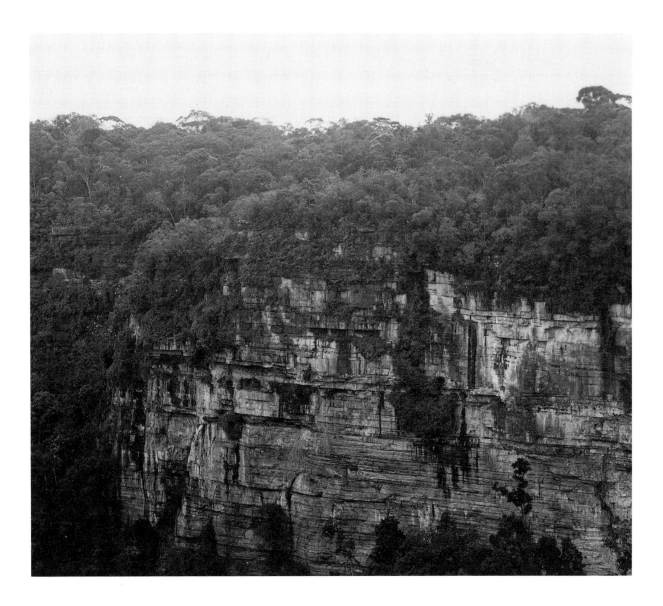

These mountains…play an important part in…mythology.

There is apparently a belief in some sort of afterlife. Cubeos have a tradition that the souls of the dead reside in or near a series of sandstone caverns on one of the open savannah areas between the headwaters of the Río Kuduyarí and the Río Cubiyú, known as the Yapobodá ("savannah of the deer").

P.H. Allen (1947)

# Quartzitic cave

*Yapobodá, Río Kuduyarí, Vaupés*

Indians believe that these caves are the homes of ancestors who can leave the caves at will and wander far and wide. Naturally, they are invisible, but some of the shamans maintain that their own souls, which leave the body during intoxication from "vine of the soul", can see and converse with these wandering beings who tell them about life in the caves. According to the natives, some of the caves have crude designs or images of animals on the walls which are believed to have had a supernatural origin.

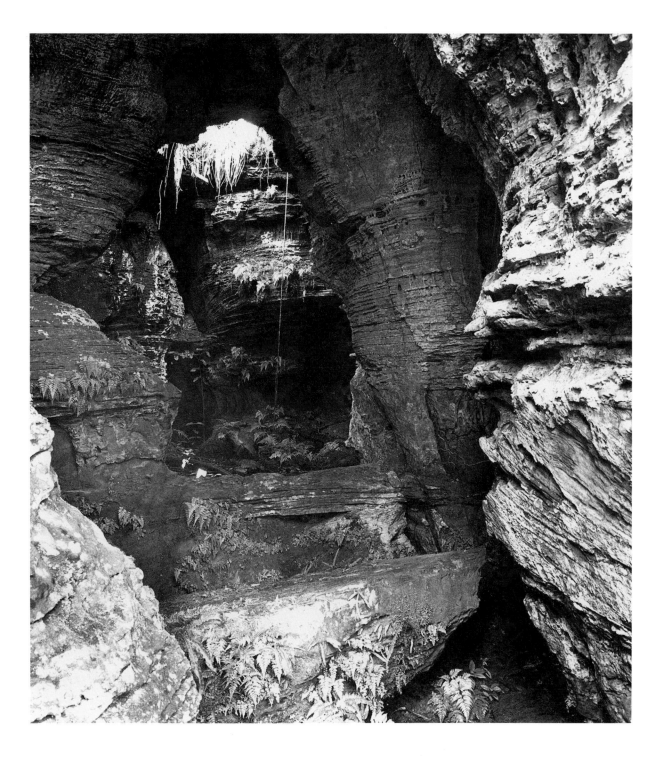

…souls of the dead reside in…sandstone caverns…

The crevasses and falls are sacred places for the numerous groups of Indians who live in the region. They are places where the celestial anaconda snake left his traces in his travels to the headwaters of the rivers in order to establish the dwelling localities of all of the tribes: Mirañas, Yukunas, Tanimukas, Makunas, Barasanas and Tatuyos.

C.A. Domínguez, (1987)

# Deep quartzitic chasm

*Cerro Castillo, Río Apaporis, Caquetá*

The numerous crevasses in the quartzitic mountains scattered throughout the Colombian Amazonia fill the Indians with fear. Some are very deep and of curious shapes, and it is in these that dangerous monsters are believed to dwell. The most harmful, say the payés, are those that can make themselves invisible but often sing or shriek, uttering shrill cries that reverberate with weird echoes against the walls.

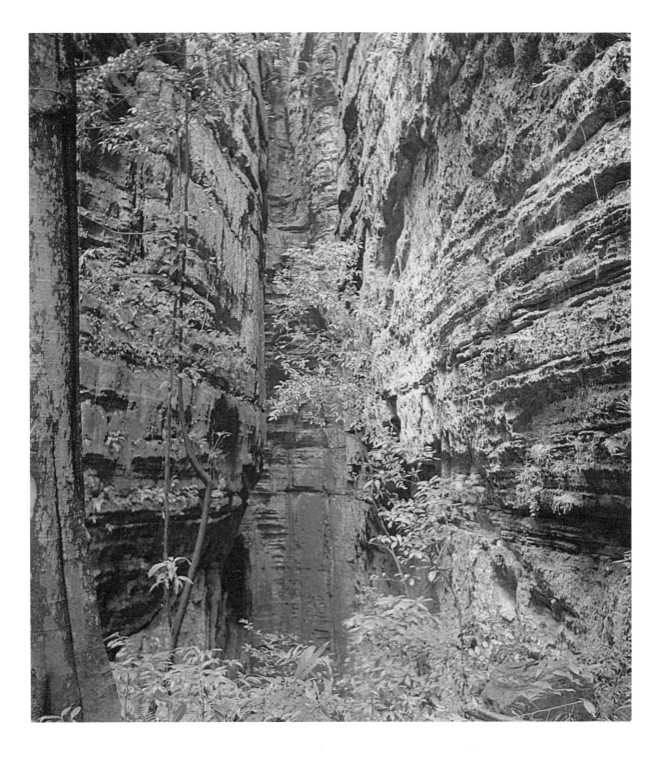

…crevasses…are sacred places…

...any extraordinary rock is
always said to be inhabited by
monstrous animals.

E.F. Imthurn (1883)

# Typical eroded quartzitic mountain tops

*Savannah Kañendá, Río Kubiyú, Vaupés*

The geological devastation of the soft quartzitic mountain tops
has left literally hundreds of bizarrely eroded rocks, many of
which are suggestive of animals. It is natural that these are
interpreted as works of spiritual forces and associated in the
Indian mind with supernatural activity.

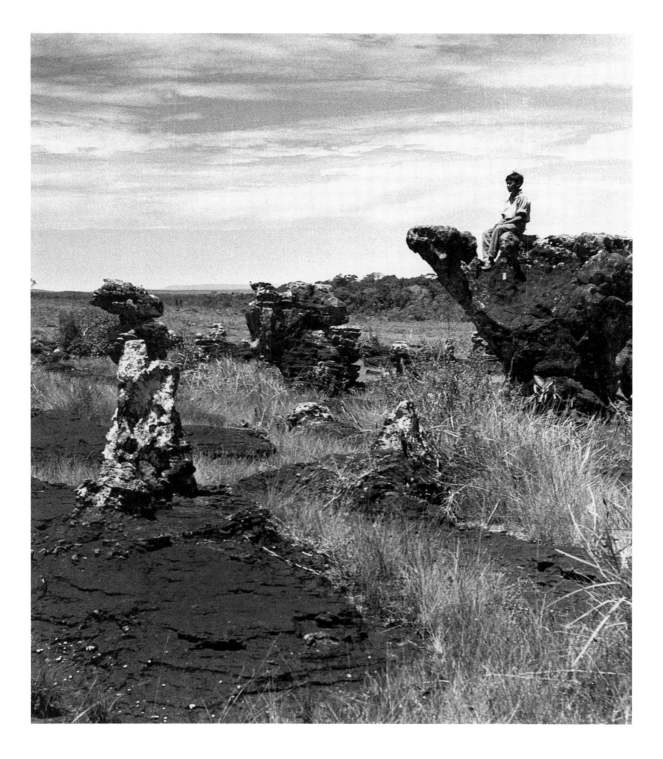

…any extraordinary rock…(is) inhabited by monstrous animals.

The religion is a primitive, little-understood belief in forest and water spirits, most of which are believed to be harmful and which must be variously propitiated.

P.H. Allen (1947)

# The great stone spirit face

*Falls of Jerijerimo, Río Apaporis, Vaupés*

In the long cliff-enclosed and strangely silent tunnel through which the waters of the Río Apaporis must pass after tumbling over the thunderous Falls of Jerijerimo, there is, sculptured by natural causes over the centuries, the face of a god. Jerijerimo is a sacred place to the Taiwano Indians who believe that the sculpture was put there by the gods to indicate that they were still in charge of the waters and that this passage was especially sacred to them.

Below the Falls of Jerijerimo there is a canyon four or five miles long before the waters widen out into the usual river. Above this long canyon there is an interesting savannah full of unusual plants. Our native paddlers preferred to meet us with all our baggage at the end of the canyon, because their Taiwano payé told them never to look upon the face of the god who lived below the waterfall. We paddled down through the canyon alone; the boys met us at its end.

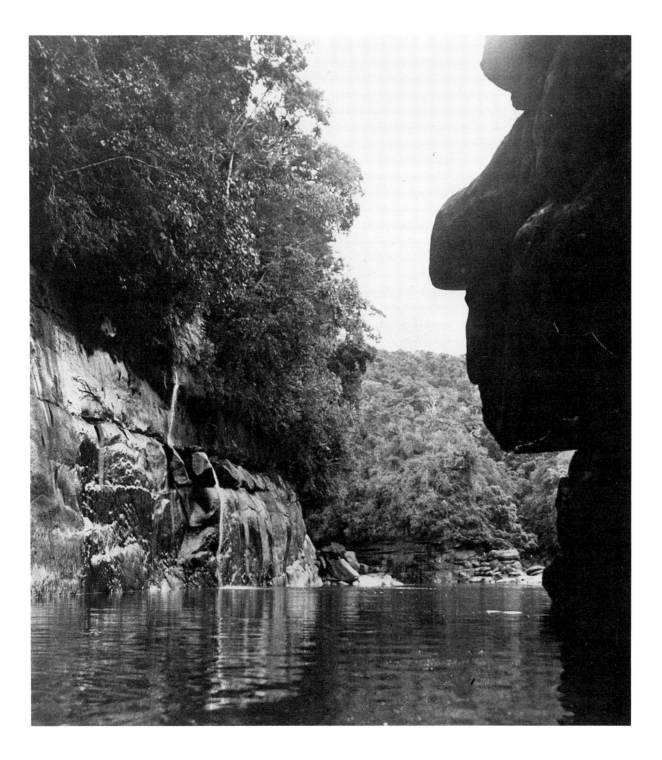

The religion is a…little-understood belief in spirits…

It is no myth that the dorsal surface of a crocodilian has a definite resemblance to a log or a lichen-covered stone.

P. Cutright (1940)

# Crocodile stone

*Yapobodá, Río Kuduyarí, Vaupés*

There can be no question that this long quartzitic stone, with a rough surface resembling a crocodile and an end with what appears to be a head and eyes, would enter into local superstition. Many oddly shaped rocks or cliffs that resemble animals are natural and, from the Indian's point of view, logical representations of animal spirits.

Kubeo Indians assured us that this stone image represented a crocodile that disobeyed the spirits controlling the rivers by venturing onto the savannah to see what life might be there; he was punished by being forced to remain forever far from a river.

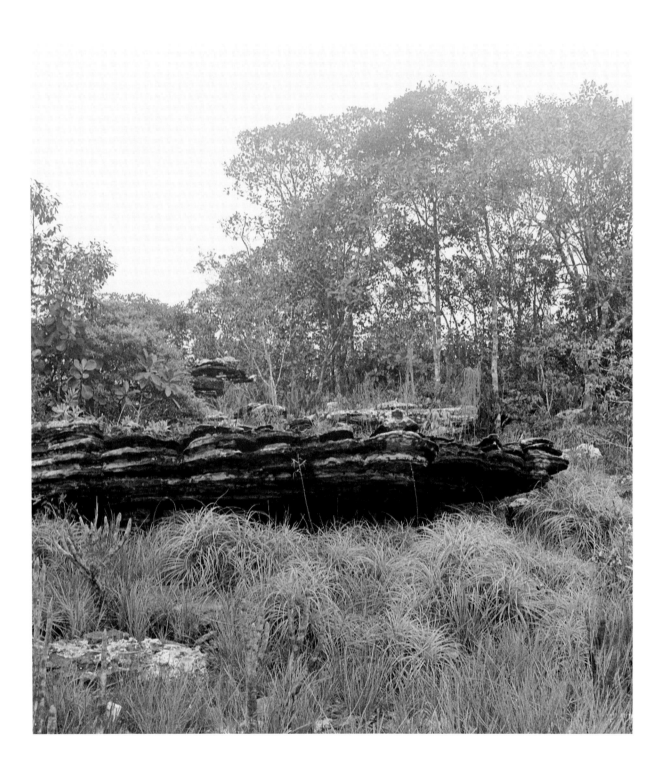

a crocodilian has a…resemblance to a…stone.

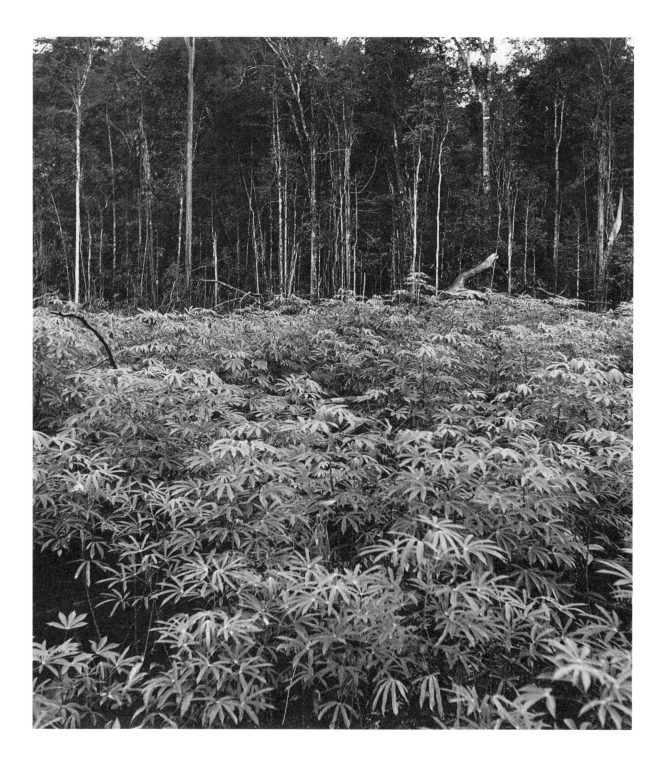

Parturition takes place in the…manioc garden.

Parturition takes place in
the woman's manioc garden.
A woman is active until the
moment her labour begins.
I have seen a pregnant woman
leave for her manioc garden
behaving as though it were an
ordinary gardening day and
return later in the afternoon with
a new-born baby.... A woman
about to give birth must alert
her husband so that he will not
leave the house or do anything
strenuous that would interfere
magically with the delivery
and the safety of the infant.

I. Goldman (1963)

# A field of manioc

*Río Kananarí, Vaupés*

Cultivation of manioc is done exclusively by the women in the
Vaupés. They are referred to by the shamans as "food mothers".
The edible tubers—the staff of life throughout the Amazon—are
said to be their children. Whether the prevalent custom of giving
birth in the manioc garden is the result of this curious shamanistic
belief or *vice versa* is difficult to explain.

Infants are bathed often and in
circumstances that are pleasurable
...[the mother] finds it a welcome
interruption from arduous and
monotonous chores.... The head-
man or shaman [is] responsible
for blowing over the river with
tobacco smoke and chanting away
its dangers.... The spell that is
chanted as the river is "blown"
refers to the anacondas, asking
them not to notice the people who
are bathing.... The river anaconda
and other water creatures...are
enraged at the birth of a child
and must be made to leave.

I. Goldman (1963)

## Kubeo mother bathing a very young infant

*Soratama, Río Apaporis, Amazonas*

A new-born baby is bathed usually as soon as the mother has
brought the child to the maloca from the manioc field. Following
the bathing, the mother paints red dots on the child's face and
body. This curious procedure is done to make the baby resemble
the jaguar, thus assuring protection of the child from this animal
of such importance in Indian superstitions and religion. It is also
believed to be necessary to make the infant a member of the
human race.

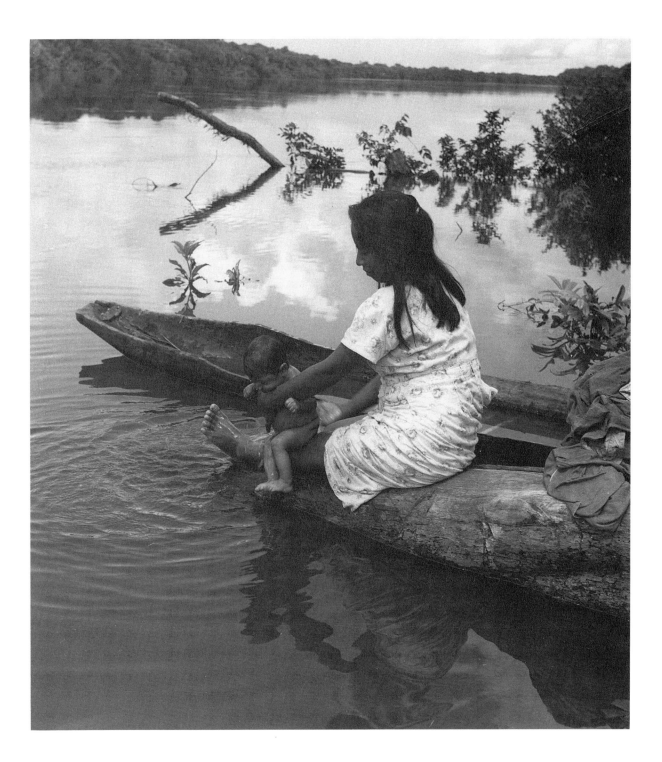

...the anaconda...(is) enraged at the birth of a child...

The wilderness background of
the contraceptive is interesting
because it is one of the few jungle
drugs whose clinical effectiveness
we have been able to check with
reasonable accuracy in the field....
The ferreting out of its secrets
presented unusual obstacles,
for its manufacture is not only
shrouded by the veils of witchcraft
and superstitious ritual, but is part
of one aspect of primitive people
which is even harder to penetrate
than the black magic of the witch
doctors. It is a "woman thing."

R. Gill (1940)

# An abundant aroid of the savannahs

*Yapobodá, Río Kuduyarí, Vaupés*

This abundant plant (*Philodendron dyscarpium*, of the Araceae or
Aroid Family) growing on the rocks of quartzitic savannahs is
said to be the "best" of the three species of aroids valued by the
Indians as contraceptives. It is reportedly sometimes used by
women who wish to punish a husband whom they do not love by
denying him children.

It has been suggested that phallic symbolism has been involved
with the evolution of the contraceptive use of the several aroid
species because of the shape of the inflorescence.

Nothing is known of the chemical constituents of this abundant
species. The obvious phallic symbolism of the erect spadix may be
responsible for its native use, but the employment of several other
members of the same family for the same purpose in the Colombian Amazon suggests the advisability of chemical and pharmacological evaluation.

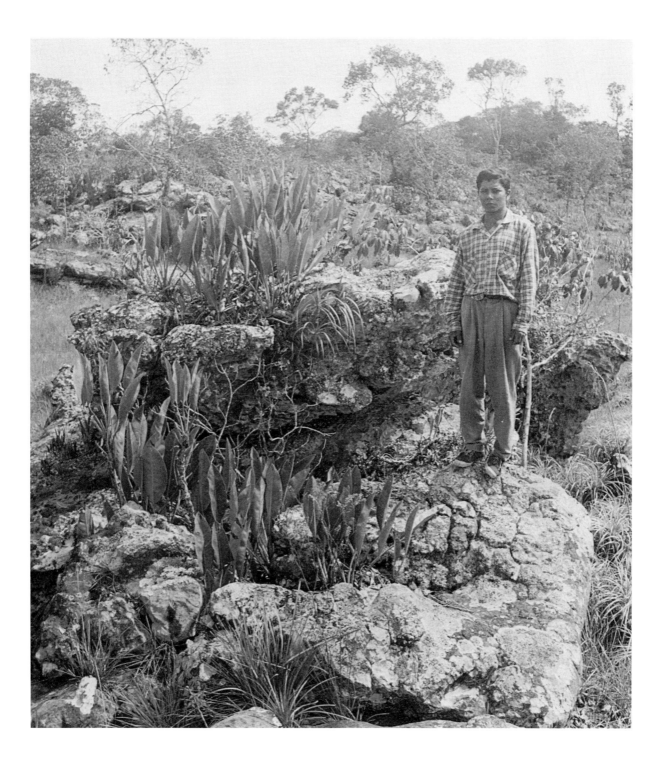

...shrouded by the veils of witchcraft...

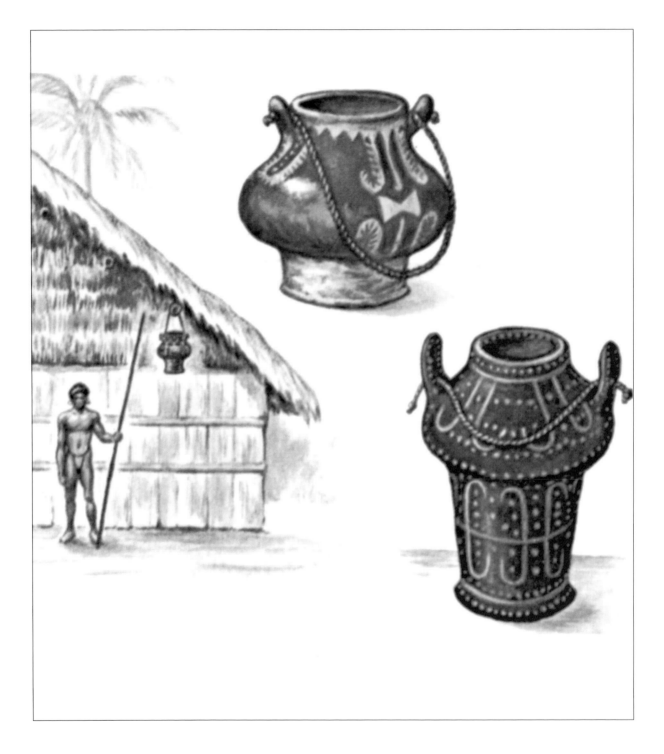

…always the same bellied form…

The caapi pot has always the same bellied form and painted with yellow designs and a deep red background.... It is never washed but is redecorated from time to time.

T. Koch Grünberg (1909)

## The sacred caapi pot

*All Tukanoan tribes, Vaupés*

The ceremonial caapi pot is said to represent the female body. While the designs may vary somewhat, they always seem to have circular or oval motifs, the significance of which is obscure. The invariable basic red suggests a mystical connotation. The vessel always hangs outside the maloca protected from the rain under the eaves in the right corner of the roof as one enters the main door.

During the manufacture of a caapi pot, which will be passed down from generation to generation, strict ritual, involving traditional chanting by the shaman, controls every step of the operation.

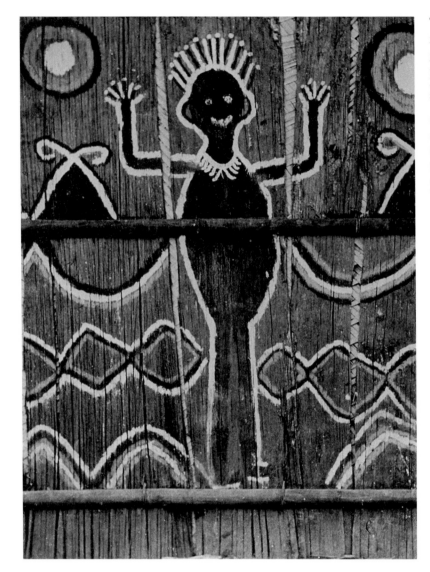

The Tukano sometimes cover the fronts of their houses with large geometric or representational paintings executed with mineral pigments on the walls of bark. When asked about the significance of these paintings they answered simply: "These are the things we see when we take yajé, they are the *gahpi-ghori*"— the yajé images.

G. Reichel-Dolmatoff (1972)

…the *gahpi-ghori*, the yajé images…

# Decoration on walls of a Makuna house

*Río Piraparaná, Vaupés*

Wall decorations always have symbolic meaning to the Indian. Usually the designs have their origin in the visions experienced during intoxication with caapi, but often, as in the case of the frequent circular motifs representing the sun and moon, they are borrowed from the petroglyphs which are believed to have had a supernatural origin.

The Indians associate all of the petroglyphs in this region with their own mythology.... The sun and moon are supernatural beings in traditional Tukanoan mythology.

F. Trupp (1981)

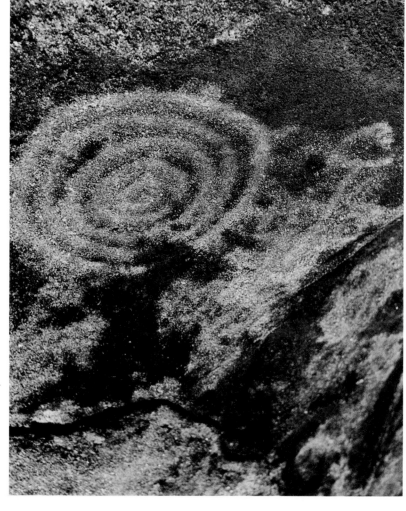

...supernatural beings in ...mythology.

## Petroglyph of the sun

*Río Piraparaná, Vaupés*

The sun and moon are considered to represent supernatural beings and, as such, play extremely significant roles in aboriginal mythology. The ancient petroglyphs abundant in the Vaupés frequently represent these important elements of native religious beliefs by concentric rings or circles.

Then there are the rock carvings...
archaic yet extraordinarily alive....
Many of the figures portrayed sun
and moons.... What is the significance of these drawings?

B. Moser and D. Tayler (1965)

# Barasanas examining sacred petroglyphs

*Río Piraparaná, Vaupés*

The Río Piraparaná in the Vaupés is one of the richest areas for
petroglyphs. There is one locality, at the head of an impassable
rapids, where there are many of these engravings within a hundred feet of rock face. The Barasanas, who must stop to portage
their canoes at this point, believe that this artistry represents one
of the spots where their supernatural beings once dwelt and
made the images before the advent of the first human beings on
the earth.

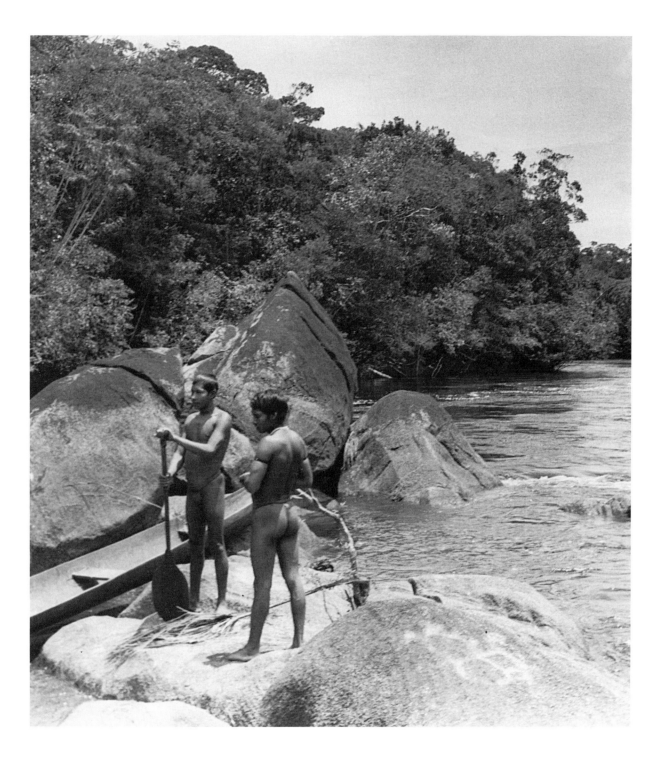

...archaic yet extraordinarily alive...

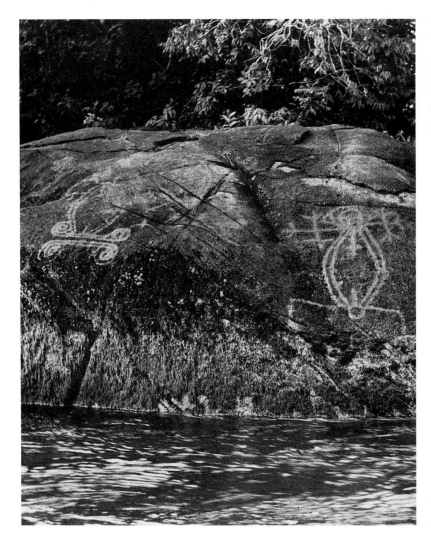

Several landmarks in the northwest Amazon are pointed out... as the place where mankind had its origin...All of them have this in common: they are huge rocks and boulders...at large waterfalls, and most of them are covered with ancient petroglyphs.

G. Reichel-Dolmatoff (1975)

...huge rocks...at large waterfalls...are covered with ancient petroglyphs.

## A common motif in rock engravings

*Yavareté, Río Vaupés, Vaupés*

In the vicinity of Yavareté on the Río Vaupés there are many petroglyphs. Some of them are located on rocks bordering tremendous rapids, and it is difficult to understand how Indians could create such time-demanding chipping on extremely hard granite rocks under these supposedly dangerous conditions. The mystery of their creation by people with only stone tools stuns the imagination and allows us to understand why today's Indians believe in the supernatural origin of these works of art.

Perhaps the most impressive specimens [of petroglyphs] are... found in the equatorial forests of Colombia, where they represent a living element in the culture of the...tribes.... The Indians... associate them with various concepts in their magical and religious beliefs.

F. Trupp (1981)

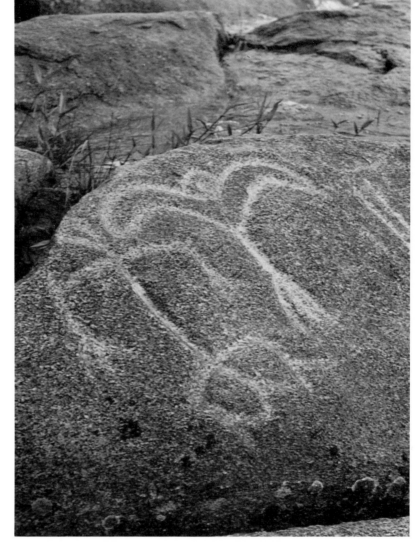

...a living element in the culture of the...tribes...

## Petroglyphs on granite

*Yavareté, Río Vaupés, Vaupés*

Many of the figures most abundant in the petroglyphs of the Vaupés represent, it is believed, supernatural beings with wings. Part of this use of wings may be the result of the experiences of ancient Indians who made the engravings—experiences of flying through the air, a very frequent initial symptom of intoxication with hallucinogens.

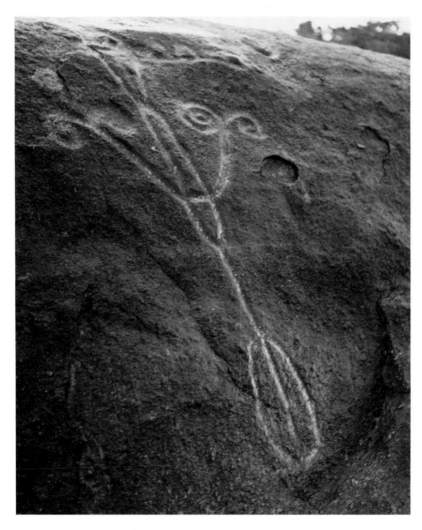

It is thought that some motifs, which appear again and again on stones and rock faces, were created under the influence of hallucinogens.

F. Trupp (1981)

...created under the influence of hallucinogens.

# Common petroglyph motif

*Rapids of Naná, Río Piraparaná, Vaupés*

Many of the most common petroglyphs are believed to be based on geometric figures "seen" under the influence of hallucinogenic plants such as caapi or yakee. At least, the Indians describe them as things they "see" during the intoxications, and the payés appear to agree to this interpretation of the figures. If this be true, it argues for the great age of the use of hallucinogens, since no knowledge of what Indians made these petroglyphs nor how old they are has been obtained. Many depict phallism suggesting fertility and procreation.

The petroglyphs are about evenly divided between geometric and naturalistic forms.... The naturalistic forms include a cross section of the modern fauna of South America....

I. Rouse (1949)

...a cross section of the modern fauna...

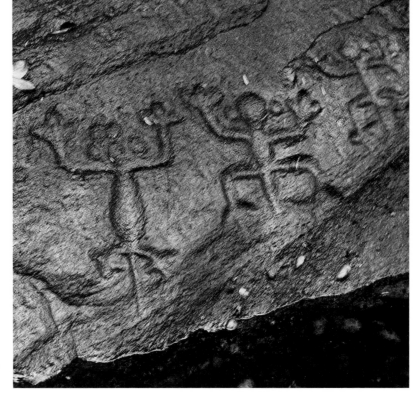

## Petroglyphs depicting animals

*Río Apaporis, Vaupés*

Almost all of the rocks in the vicinity of the more than two dozen major waterfalls or rapids in the Vaupés have rock engravings, depicting usually mythical figures. One of the surprising aspects of Indian life is the native familiarity with the stories, told from father to son, of the supernatural origin of these petroglyphs.

Many of the Indians believe that they indicate places sacred to the Master of Animals. In the Río Apaporis, depictions of animals are extremely rare. The Makunas state that the petroglyphs pictured here represent frogs. They recite the story that, at the beginning of creation, frogs were large and powerful animals, but that they were so overbearing with respect to all other animals that the Master of Animals decided to make them insignificant, lower than the fish and snakes, and that never again could they live either totally in the water or on land far from water.

...the large communal houses in which they live represent the universe: the roof is the sky, the men's door is...in the east, where the sun rises and the women's door...is in the west where the sun sets; the walls...are the edges of the world. Shamans see the house like this, as do other men, when under the effects of yajé.

S. Hugh-Jones (1979)

# Makuna round house

*Río Popeyaká, Amazonas*

Like so many other aspects of life, the large, circular maloca or house characteristic of the Makuna tribe is so constructed that it is believed to represent the universe. The main posts that support the thatched roof are the mountains supporting the sky; the smaller posts are interpreted as representing the descendents of the original sacred anaconda that came from the depths and became a human being. The beautifully fashioned roof represents the world, and the apical ridge signifies the limits of the universe itself, whilst the floor represents the earth.

The central part of the maloca is reserved for sacred dances, gatherings and meetings supervised by the payés. Each of the numerous family groups living in this communal house has a section around the inner periphery, where family life goes on.

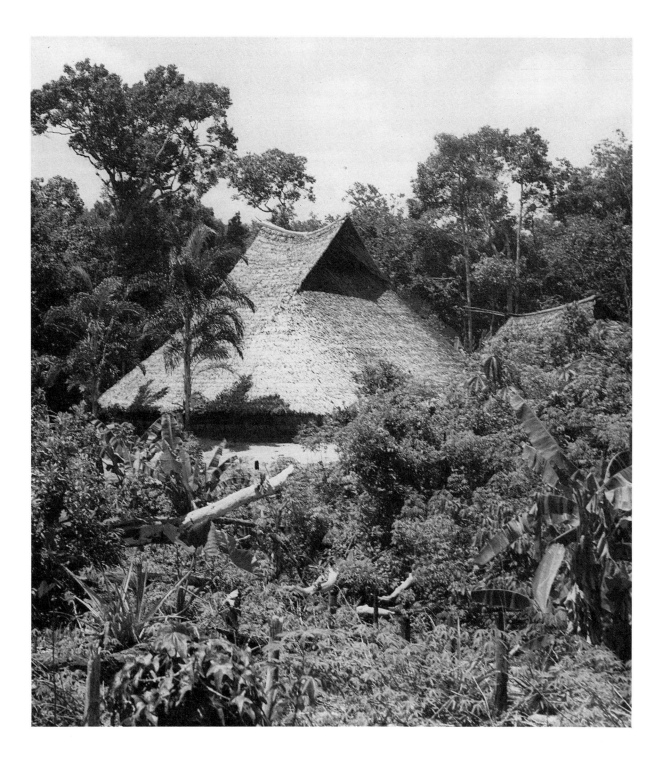

…the large houses…represent the universe…

...it has been possible to demonstrate the importance of the Indians' mythology and magico-religious symbolism...in the construction of a building, the choice of the site, the arrangement of the settlement, the place allocated to the individual families in a communal dwelling and also the artistic decoration of their homes.

F. Trupp (1981)

# Rectangular communal house

*Río Kananarí, Vaupés*

Many of the large communal houses in the Vaupés are the homes of up to eight or ten families. Each family group has a small area along the inner periphery of the enormous building, each with its hammocks and slow fire. The central part of the house is clear of habitations, reserved for the frequent ceremonial dances attended usually by many neighbouring tribal members, some of whom walk or paddle long distances to attend the festivals which often last for several days.

It is the medicine man or shaman who officiates at these ceremonies and whose advice and control has directed construction of the houses and who, in fact, "consecrates" the structure and the paintings of mythological figures that frequently adorn the outer walls of the buildings.

The rectangular maloca is typical of the Taiwanos and related tribes.

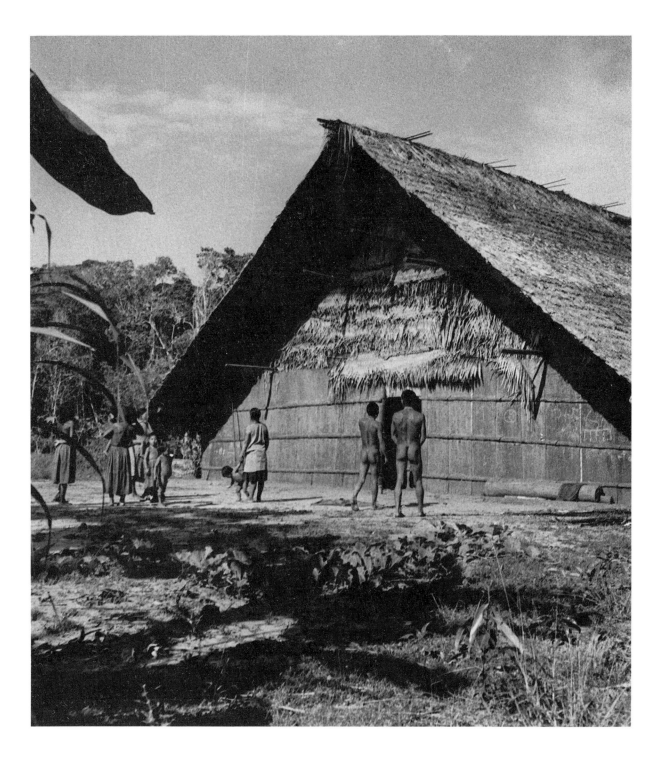

…the importance of…mythology and religious symbolism…

The central area [of the maloca] is associated with the exclusive male society and with sacred, ritual activities, whereas the periphery is the domain of family life, women and profane activities such as cooking.

S. Hugh-Jones (1979)

# The interior of a maloca

*Río Kananarí, Vaupés*

The central portion of every Indian house or maloca—the large round ones or the rectangular types—is the area reserved for the payés and the activities under their control and supervision. It is spacious and always kept scrupulously clean and well swept. It is here that the coca is prepared, an activity indicative of the once semi-sacred position of this narcotic which, however, is today a daily, profane element of male life.

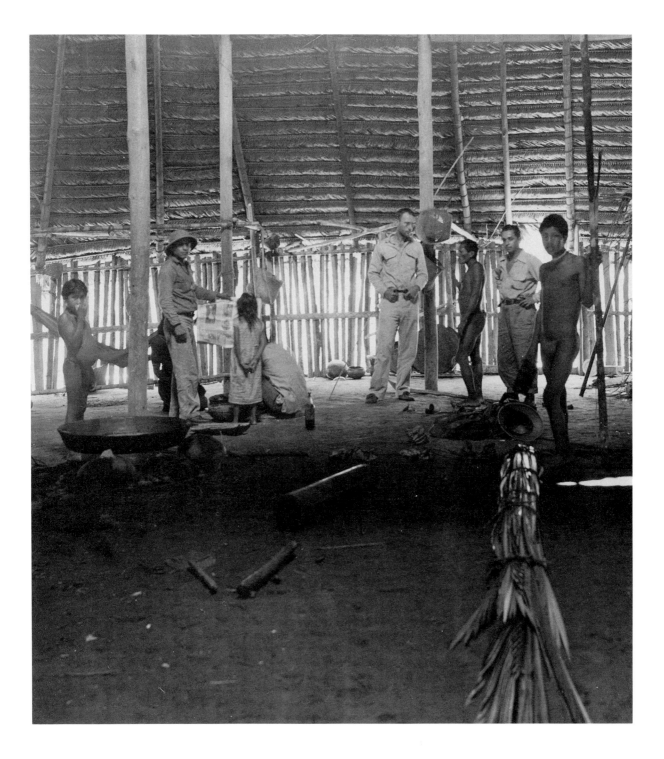

The central area…[for] sacred activities,…the periphery… [for] profane activities…

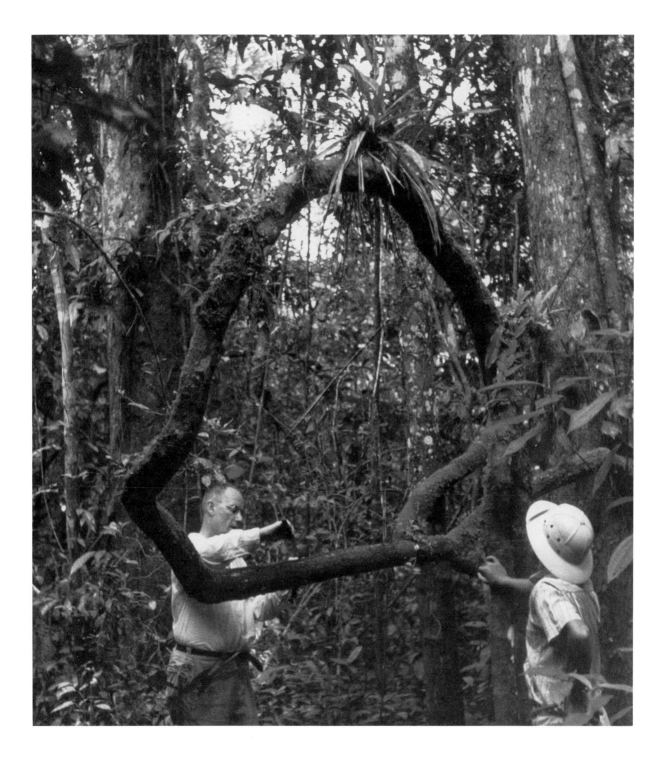

...a treasured hereditary possession.

The most important poison is the curare...The complicated recipe is a treasured hereditary possession.

T. Whiffen (1915)

# A plant of great importance in modern medicine

*Río Loretoyacu, Amazonas*

*Chondrodendron tomentosum* is the source of an alkaloid (tubocurarine), known for its relaxant or paralyzant activity on skeletal muscle. It and one or two of its semi-synthetic derivatives are of value as adjuncts in anesthesia for the production of muscle relaxation in various surgical procedures.

Native hunters prefer older plants which apparently are richer in the active principle. Since collecting the bark and roots naturally tends to kill these slow-growing lianas, this species of the westernmost Amazonian forests of Colombia, Ecuador and Peru is becoming rarer each year, posing a problem for the commercial production of the curare syrup for medical purposes.

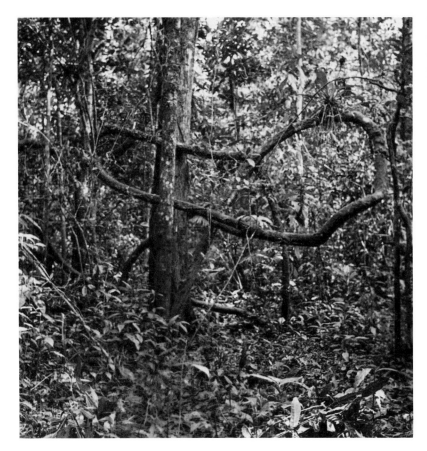

There was nothing whereof I was more curious than to finde out the true remedies of these poisoned arrows...

Sir Walter Ralegh (1595)

There is nothing whereof I was more curious

## A minor species of *Chondrodendron*

*Ucursique, Putumayo*

There are eight or nine species of Chondrodendron native to Colombia, Ecuador, Peru and Brazil. The Indian curare specialists prefer *Chondrodendron tomentosum*, but some of the other species may be utilised when this major source is not easily at hand. Those who prepare the arrow poison are quick to identify the several species, even at a distance in the forest, because of differences in growth habit, bark characteristics and other often intangible peculiarities.

The curare prepared commercially in Colombia, Ecuador and Peru as a source of the medicinally valuable d-tubocurarine is almost invariably *Chondrodendron tomentosum*, a member of the Menispermaceae, the Moonseed Family.

How far back in time the use of these poisons collectively known as curare extends cannot be determined.... Which tribe discovered and prepared curare and how this poison lore spread over such large, pathless areas of the South American continent cannot be explained.

L. Lewin (1923)

*How far back...the use of these poisons...extends cannot be determined.*

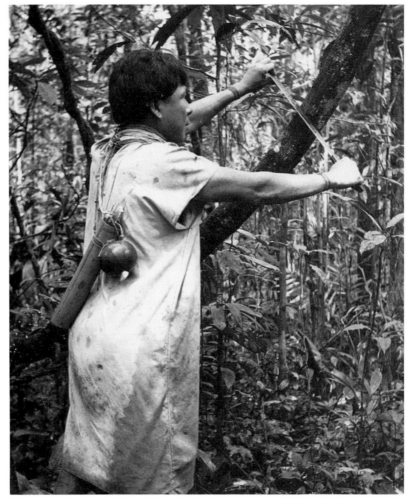

## Kofán curare-maker collecting bark

*Río Sucumbíos, Putumayo*

Knowledge of the best plant sources of curare and other factors, such as the correct time to collect the bark, the part of the liana from which it should be taken, how it should be cared for after collection, and the appropriate incantations to be made during the collection, are all part of the knowledge passed from one generation of payés to the next. They date back probably to the earliest times of curare use, an example of the precious botanical heritage of these indigenous peoples, an acquaintance with nature rapidly being lost.

He [the payé] is the poison maker
for the tribe and possesses, as a
rule...a considerable knowledge
of drugs, both curative and lethal.

T. Whiffen (1915)

# Kofán medicine man preparing curare

*Río Sucumbíos, Putumayo*

In many tribes, curare is prepared by the payé or medicine man;
in others, the poison is made by a specialist who does nothing
else. In both cases, however, a long and arduous period of
training is necessary, starting usually in an apprenticeship at an
early age. An extraordinary acquaintance with plants is naturally
required, but in most cases, strict fasting from certain foods is
demanded, and long and intricate incantations must be recited to
insure a final product of outstanding toxicity.

The Kofáns are probably the tribe in the northwest Amazonia
with the most knowledge of curare-plants. They prepare many
kinds of the poison, each with great care and elaborate taboos of
special diets and chants to make the poison effective. Are these
medicine men not worth our attention before they and their
knowledge are lost?

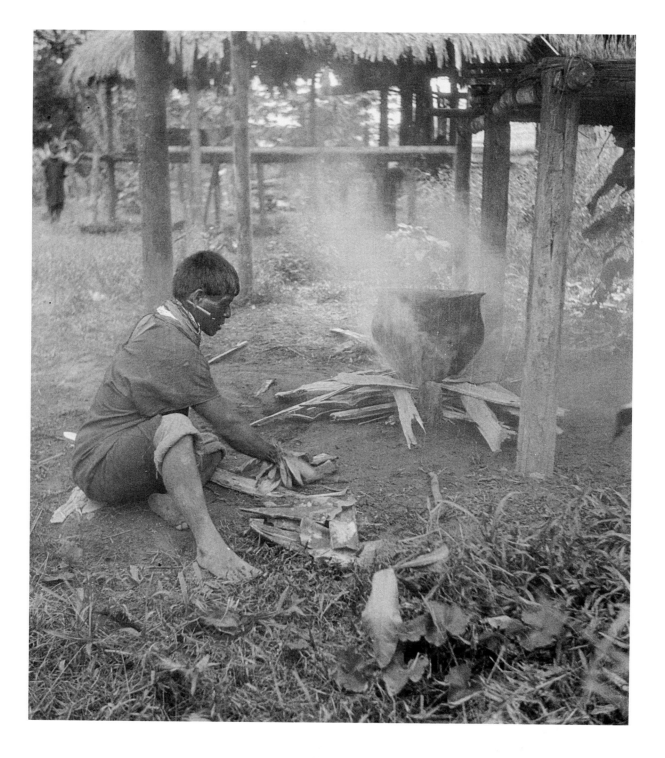

…a considerable knowledge of drugs,…curative and lethal.

He has prepared his deadly
weapons, making his arrows
fiery shafts.

The Holy Bible, Psalms vii, 13

# Kofán payé anointing darts
# with finished curare

*Río Sucumbíos, Putumayo*

Poisoning of arrows for hunting and warfare has been practiced by primitive societies on almost every continent. Different toxic plants were utilized. A reference that may be interpreted as referring to poisoned arrows appears in the Bible. The Hebrews, at the time of the Psalms, apparently did not have arrow poisons, but they undoubtedly knew that their neighbours, particularly the Greeks, did anoint arrows with poisonous substances.

The greatest number of species used as basic ingredients of curare and its many additives which may or may not have synergistic effects are employed in the Colombian Amazon.

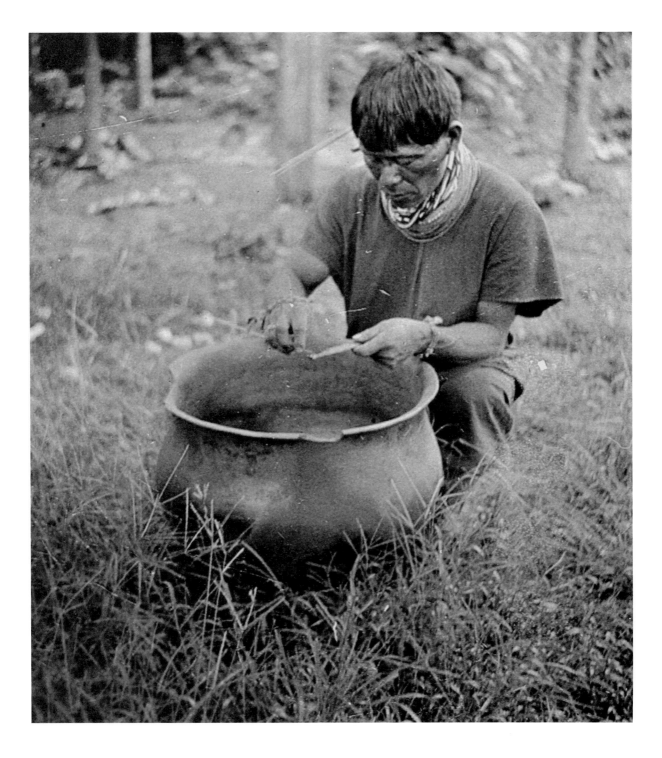

...making his arrows fiery shafts.

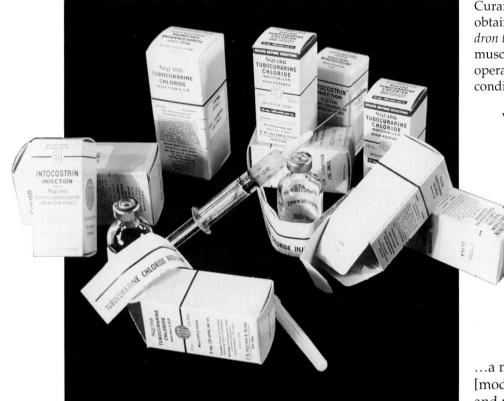

Curare [tubocurarine chloride], obtained mainly from *Chondrodendron tomentosum*, is used as a muscle relaxant in surgical operations and in neurological conditions.

V.H. Heywood, *et al.* (1978)

...a muscle relaxant in [modern] surgical operations and neurological conditions..

# A modern medicine from an ancient Amazonian plant, Tubocurarine

A convincing argument for the urgency of ethnobotanical conservation is the example of curare. Known as a preparation primarily for hunting in tropical South America for more than three centuries and often reported—frequently in greatly exaggerated terms—by the early chroniclers, it was not until the 1930s that the poison attracted the serious attention of modern medicine. It soon became evident that extracts from this aboriginal product could be employed by medical and pharmacological experts to relax muscles in surgical operations and other procedures.

How many similarly outstanding discoveries may result from examination of aboriginal knowledge of the properties of bioactive plants?

The act of preparing this poison is not considered as a common one; the savage may shape his bow, fasten the barb on the point of his arrow, and make his other implements of destruction either lying in his hammock or in the midst of his family; but, if he has to prepare the *wourali* poison, many precautions are supposed to be necessary.

C. Waterton (1825)

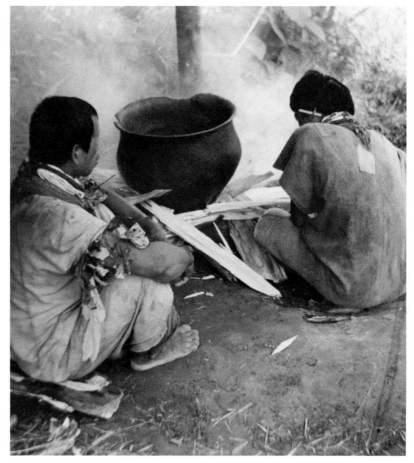

...many precautions are supposed to be necessary.

## Kofán payés collaborating to prepare a strong curare

*Río Sucumbíos, Putumayo*

Often, when an especially strong curare is needed or one destined for a very special purpose is to be made, certain definite practises must be followed. Amongst the Kofáns, if a curare is to be employed against human beings or large animals, two curare makers are usually involved in its preparation, and they intone the proper chants to be sure the toxic product will fulfill its purpose. One of the other skills of these several curare makers lies in their combined knowledge of the minor additive plants needed in the preparation of the final curare, whether these be plants with synergistic effects or species valued for magical effects.

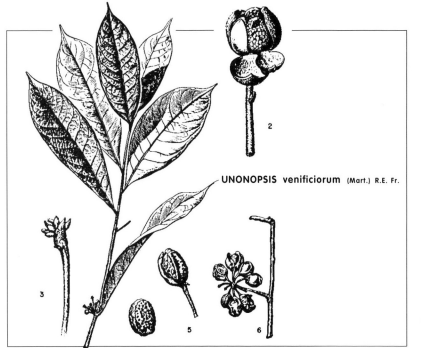

UNONOPSIS venificiorum (Mart.) R.E. Fr.

...other materials, for example... the astringent fruits of *Guatteria [Unonopsis] veneficiorum* may be added [to curare].... It grows in secondary forests along the Japurá, in the territory of the Jurí Indians who use it for curare poison.

J.B. von Spix and
C.F.P. von Martius (1824)

The Juri Indians [of the Caquetá] ...used it for a curare poison.

## An old curare plant rediscovered

*Kofáns of the Putumayo and Barasanas of the Vaupés*

Some curare plants have only recently been identified; others were reported by earlier investigators but never noted, until recent field studies.

One such curare ingredient is *Unonopsis veneficiorum* (formerly *Guatteria veneficiorum*) of the Annonaceae or Custard Apple Family. One hundred seventy years ago, a German plant explorer who collected in the Brazilian Amazon and in Colombia along the Río Caquetá as far upstream as Araracuara, found the Jurí, Miraña and other tribes using the fruits of this species as the basis of an arrow poison. No subsequent evidence of this use appeared, until recent research reported its employment in two distant localities in Colombia and Ecuador: the Barasanas of the Vaupés utilize the root and bark of the lower stem, and the Kofáns of Ecuador and the Putumayo of Colombia likewise value it in the preparation of one of their curares.

It is interesting that numerous other species of *Unonopsis* are employed in Amazonian Colombia and Peru in treating rheumatism.

The Indians claim to use a
number of plant poisons.

I. Goldman (1948)

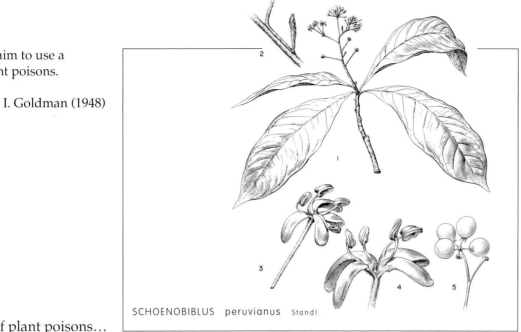

SCHOENOBIBLUS peruvianus Standl.

…a number of plant poisons…

# A Kofán curare and fish poison

*Río Sucumbíos, Putumayo*

It is well known that the Indians of the northwest Amazonia
employ many plants as basic ingredients in some of their curares.
An interesting example of such use is a plant recently found as a
source of both a curare and a fish poison: *Schoenobiblus peruvianus*
of the Thymelaeaceae or Daphne Family.

The Kofáns of Colombia and Ecuador employ the fruits and roots,
almost always without admixture, in preparing a kind of curare
used to kill birds. It is said that occasionally they may add one of
two species of *Selaginella*, a fern relative, which, so far as is known,
has no bioactive constituents. The fruits are used as a fish poison.

The Kofáns are the only Indians known to utilize this species for
these purposes. The Tikunas of the Río Loretoyacu dry and
powder the leaves to poultice persistent infected cuts and wounds
to hasten healing.

While the chemical constituents of the species have not been
analyzed, the family is rich in coumarin derivatives, the medicinal
value of which is well recognized. The range of bioactivity of these
compounds is, however, not fully appreciated at the present time.

...one of the first diagnostic characters used by the Kofáns in identifying a plant is its taste.... It is quite possible that bitterness ...led to the original discovery of the plants used for their arrow poisons. Moreover, in many cultures, bitterness has become associated with death.

A.J. Kostermans *et al.* (1969)

# A recently discovered source of curare

*Río Guamués, Putumayo, Colombia and Río Aguarico, Ecuador*

It is true that even today perhaps only a fraction of what the Amazonian Indians know about arrow-poison plants is known to modern science. This native knowledge is, in many parts, rapidly disappearing, and modern medicine and toxicology will lose a valuable store of ethnobotanical information, if more field research is not begun.

The native peoples, if properly approached and treated, are friendly, willing—even anxious—to share their knowledge, with the interested scientist. Rarely is there secrecy about their knowledge if the native is approached in a gentlemanly manner for, after all, he—especially the medicine man—is a gentleman as the most highly respected and knowledgeable man in his tribe.

Recent research has discovered a species of Lauraceae or Laurel Family, *Ocotea venenosa*, the fruits of which are an ingredient of curare amongst the Kofáns.

Several alkaloids have been isolated from this plant; they are chemically related to d-tubocurarine, the alkaloid of curare prepared from *Chondrodendron tomentosum* which is valuable in modern medicine as a muscle relaxant.

It has truly been said that the mystery of all the curares is by no means solved.

OCOTEA venenosa *Kosterm. et Pinkley*

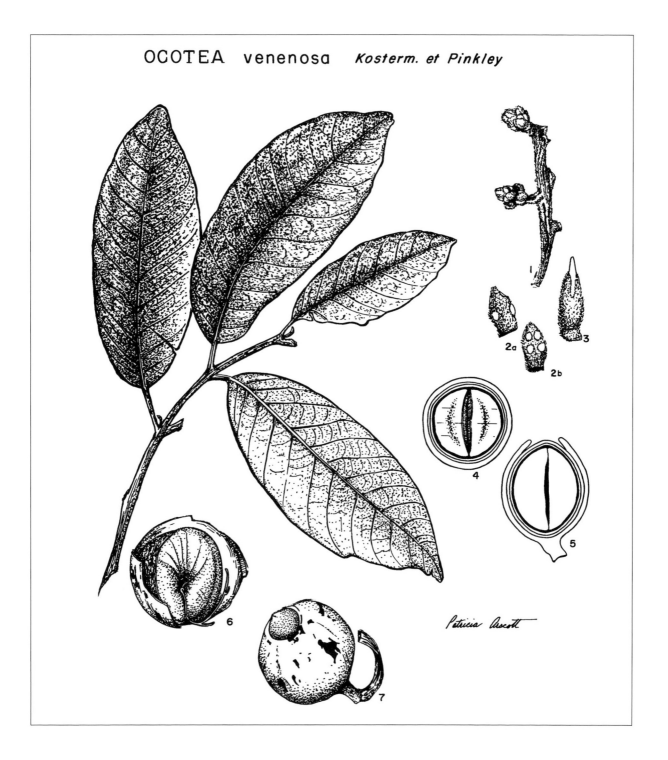

...bitterness...associated with death.

A wadding of cotton that will receive the impact of the air puff is attached to the butt of the dart. Since the wad is part of the dart when it is loaded, the Indians carry a supply of floss in a little calabash...tied to their quivers.

A. Métraux (1949)

# Fibre from the kapok tree for the darts

*Río Sucumbíos, Putumayo*

To propel the poisoned darts to the tops of the jungle trees from the long blowgun, the slender six- or eight-inch darts must have an appreciable force behind them. This is provided by applying a plug of light "cotton" from the kapok tree to the distal, non-poisoned end of the dart; the plug just fills the bore of the blowgun, so that the not-too-strong puff of the hunter is sufficiently powerful to blow the dart through the weapon and on the way to its prey.

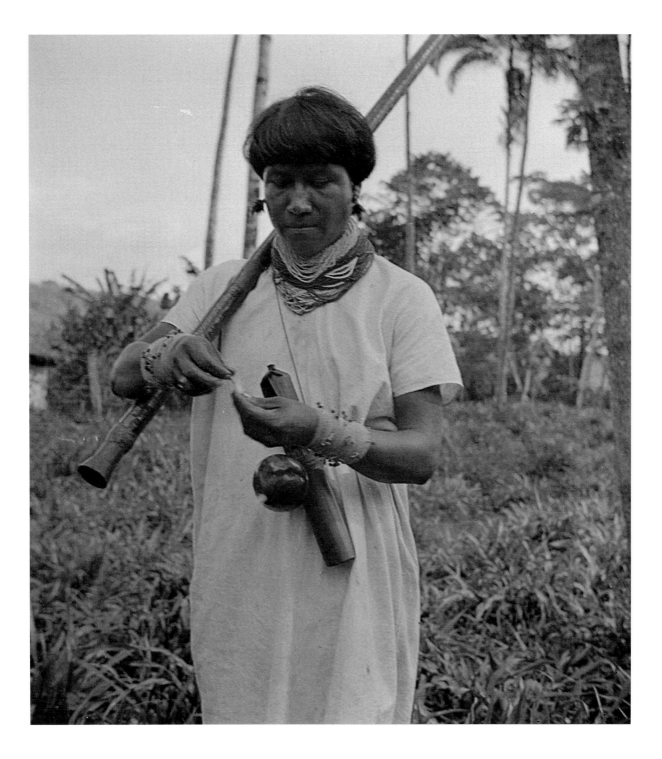

...a supply of floss in a little calabash...

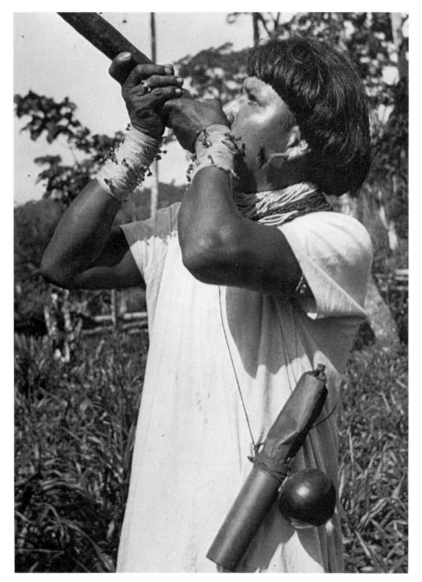

Quivers are variously made ... [often] a section of bamboo is used.

R.H. Lowie (1948)

Quivers are variously made…

# Siona hunter with bamboo quiver

*Ucursique, Putumayo*

In the Colombian Putumayo, the commonest kind of quiver is made from a piece of bamboo stem, the end of which is plugged and sealed with resin. This is the easiest type to fabricate, but it serves its purpose in holding up to 50 of the slender, poisoned darts awaiting insertion into the blowgun.

...quivers...are twilled baskets.... The bottom is made of wood or a gourd.... The outer surface is smeared with wax or pitch; sometimes...the quivers are partly covered with an additional layer of basketry with geometrical designs.

A. Métraux (1949)

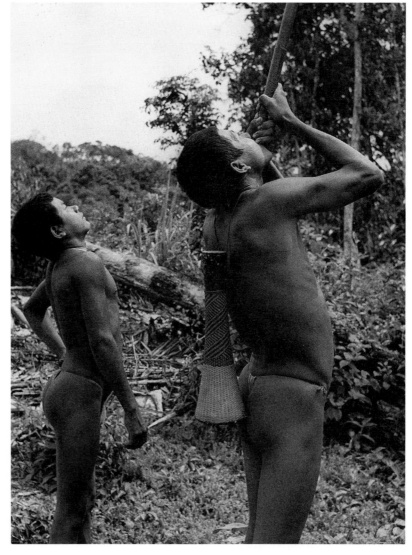

...quivers...are twilled baskets with...designs.

## Typical Tukanoan basketry quiver

*Río Piraparaná, Vaupés*

In the Colombian Amazon, there are two types of quivers in which hunters keep their poisoned darts. In the Vaupés and other parts of the region, the quivers are intricate and often decorated round baskets, sealed at one end; in the Putumayo, the bamboo type is used, In both cases, specially trained assistants of the curare-maker fabricate the quivers.

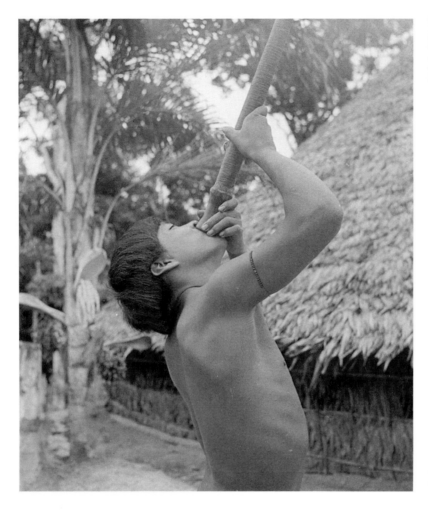

When shooting, the Indian holds the tube with both hands, palm down, close to the mouth and with the right uppermost.

A. Métraux (1949)

…the Indian holds the tube with both hands…

## A Makuna lad practicing blowgun shooting

*Río Popeyaká, Amazonas*

Boys learn how to handle the blowgun at an early age. Very often, small blowguns are made for the youngest who gradually become strong and proficient enough to shoot with the eight- or nine-foot instrument which adults handle with extreme dexterity. To hold such a long and heavy tube still with both hands at the mouthpiece end requires great strength which only practice can provide. Another aspect of blowgun use demanding long practice is the ability to walk quietly through the dense underbrush of the forest without entanglement of this long weapon in the many vines and branches.

The arrow poison, coupled with the blowgun, was a marvelous solution found by the Indians... Faced with...capturing his fleeting prey in thickets and jungles which hindered his movements and reduced visibility, the Indian had to search for something that killed without noise and without poisoning the flesh of his catch, that killed or paralyzed almost instantaneously, that carried the darts some distance but did not cause the animal to bleed, lest the effect of the curare be reduced....

E. Pérez-Arbeláez (1959)

...a marvellous solution found by the Indians...

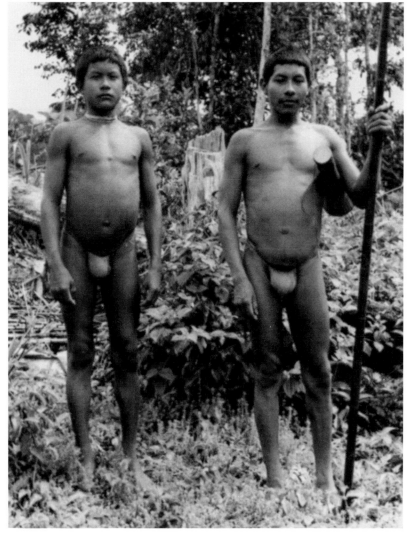

# Young and expert Makú hunters

*Río Piraparaná, Vaupés*

The blowgun, known locally as *bodaquera* or *cerbatana*, is an ingenious invention. For hunting in the dark depths of the forest it is, in many respects, superior to the shotgun because of its silence. Expert hunters can blow the delicate poisoned darts to great distances without a sound. In this way, birds, monkeys and other animals are not frightened away and frequently several or many of the desired prey can be shot and fall to the ground.

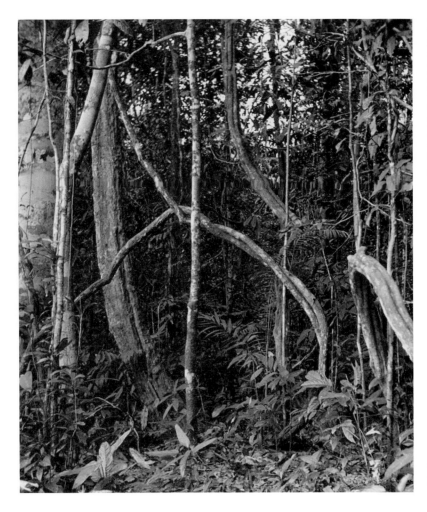

Rotenone was first known as a mysterious and unidentified fish poison or barbasco of the deep jungles of South America. There the natives collected the roots of certain forest plants and utilized them to poison small streams or pools, thereby causing the fish to float to the surface where they are easily collected.

R.W. Schery (1972)

Rotenone...a mysterious and unidentified fish poison...

## The most potent fish poison—a forest liana

*Río Karaparaná, Amazonas*

Species of plants with ichthyotoxic potential are numerous, but in Colombian Amazonia most use is made of the bark of several forest lianas of the Leguminosae or Bean Family: *Lonchocarpus Nicou*, *L. utilis* and *L. Urucu*. These are common in the region but not abundant in many other parts of Amazonia. In some localities, the natives cultivate at least one species of this genus.

The active constituent in these lianas is rotenone, now employed in the agricultural areas of the United States as a biodegradable insecticide.

Fishing with *barbasco* poison... is a special event in which the payé plays an important role by invoking *Vai-mahsé* [Master of Game Animals] and also by "opening a path" so that the poison flows and is effectively diluted in the water.

G. Reichel-Dolmatoff (1971)

Fishing with barbasco... is a special event....

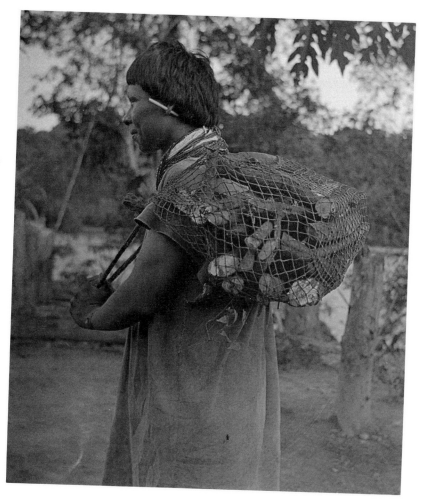

## Kofán bringing in *Lonchocarpus* fish poison

*Conejo, Río Sucumbíos, Putumayo*

When the Indians choose a vine of *Lonchocarpus*, usually one of great age which they consider to be "stronger in poison", they may have to fell several trees to have the extensive liana fall from the crowns in which it has grown entwined. After the liana has fallen to the ground, large pieces of the trunk and sometimes the root are cut off and carried back to the maloca and stored for use. They are either debarked when the natives want to use them in fishing, or the smaller pieces are completely macerated by pounding. The bark or the crushed stems are then dragged slowly through still water in a fibre basket.

...the shaman...can make contact
with the spirit [the Lord of the
Fish] and ask him for permission
to fish.

F. Trupp (1981)

# Kofáns fishing with barbasco

*Río Guamués, Putumayo*

The fish poison—whether the stem and roots of the liana
Lonchocarpus or the leaves and stems of the shrub Phyllanthus—
must be crushed before being cast into still water or dragged
slowly through slow-flowing water. In either case, the fish are not
killed but stupefied, as the barbasco affects the function of the
gills; and they come to the surface seeking oxygen and are easily
picked up by the natives who are waiting in canoes.

This method of fishing can, of course, be practiced only in
sparsely populated regions, but indigenous peoples in both hemi-
spheres and on almost all continents have discovered numerous
plants that interfere with the respiration of fish. Tropical South
America appears to have a greater number of fish poison plants
than any other region of the world.

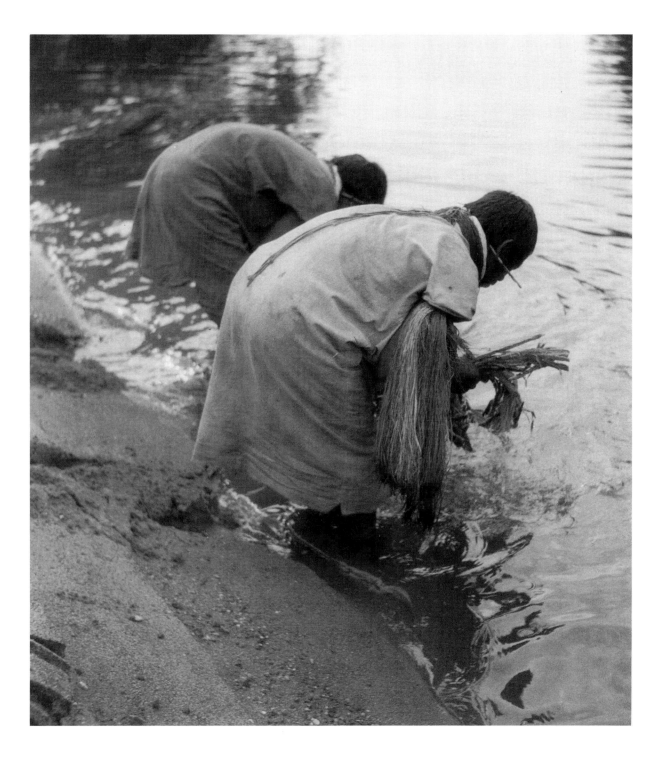

…contact with the spirit…for permission to fish.

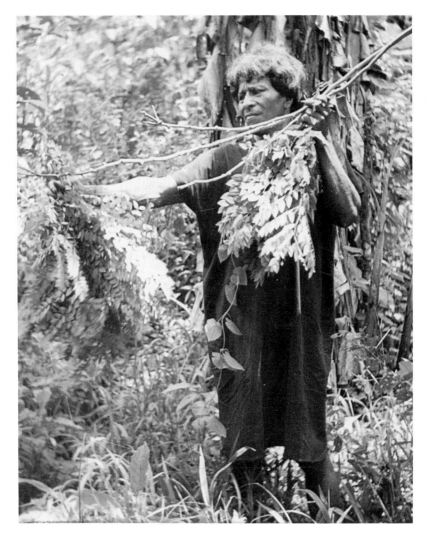

...in the clearing of the forest, the Indian will usually save from destruction any economic plant... ants will not have their nests near a *cunaparú* plant (Phyllanthus sp.), the milky juice of which is acrid and insufferably irritant, and it is for this reason that many fields contain two or three of these plants.

W.E. Roth (1924)

...in the clearing of the forest...

# One of the fish poisons of the forest

*Ucursique, Putumayo*

Most of the plants used as fish poisons are cultivated. A few, like this shrubby species of Phyllanthus are gathered from the forest. Care is taken when a patch of forest is cleared for agriculture to see that plants valued for fishing are left standing.

Alkaloids, terpenes, glycosides and other constituents have been isolated from species of this genus, but those responsible for the piscicidal activity have apparently not been defined.

The use of plant piscicides...is probably an old cultural pursuit in native South America. This historico-geographical deduction is borne out by botanical studies indicating that certain plants have not been recorded away from the precincts of man and are known only from cultivated specimens.

R.F. Heizer (1949)

...an old cultural pursuit in...native South America.

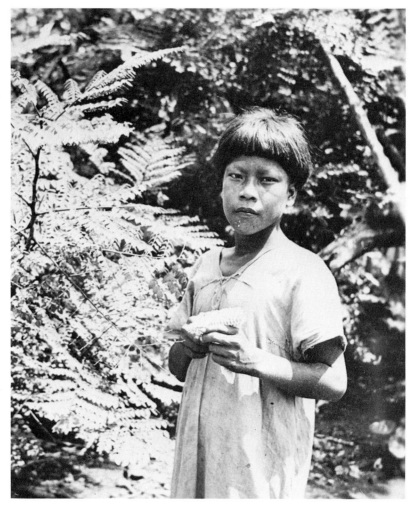

## Siona Indians and cultivated *Phyllanthus*

*Nuevo Mundo, Caquetá*

One of the commonest of the cultivated barbascos is Phyllanthus *piscatorum*. This species is unknown in the wild, usually an indication of long cultivation and use.

The leaves and branches are harvested; they rapidly regenerate from new sprouts. The harvested material is easily at hand and is crushed and thrown into still water or dragged in a bag if the water is not still; the ichthyotoxic activity begins within five or ten minutes.

The principal use of Phyllanthus
amongst the natives is in fishing....

H. García-Barriga (1974)

## Siona Indians pounding *barbasco*

*Puerto Limón, Río Caquetá, Cauca*

The word barbasco is a general term for fish poisons. One of the
favourite and most easily used barbascos consists of branches
and occasionally roots of several species of Phyllanthus of the
Spurge Family. The material must be crushed by vigorous pounding; frequently it is allowed to ferment before use. It is then
packed into a netted bag and dragged gently through the water;
within minutes, fish come to the surface for oxygen and are easily
caught.

This genus has been found to have alkaloids, terpenes and
lignans.

268

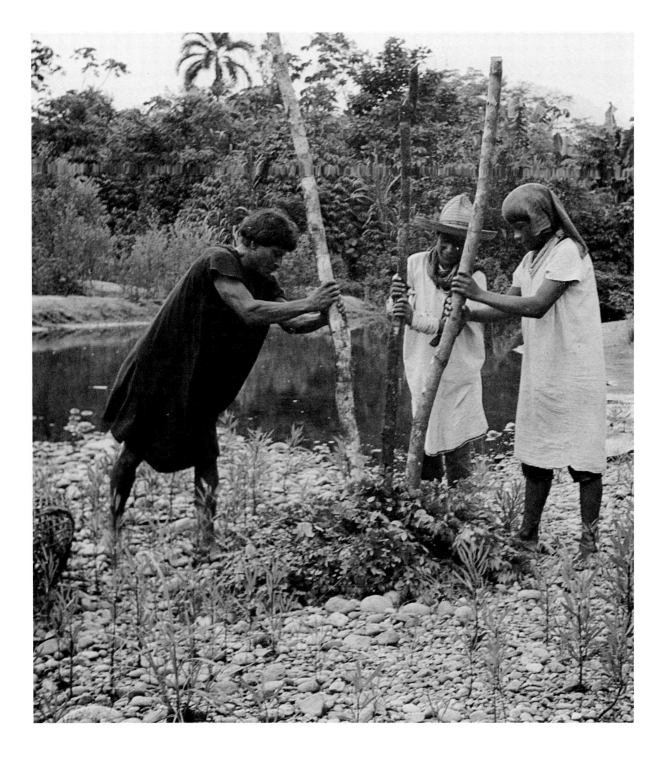

The principal use…is in fishing….

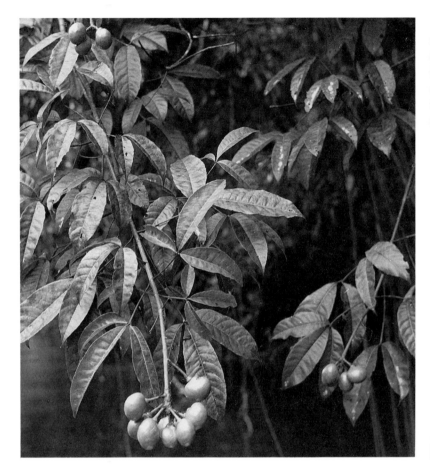

Piquiá is the name of an edible nut the pulp of which is poisonous. As a result, after it is crushed, there remains a mass which, when cast into the water, stupefies fish that float to the surface and are caught by hand or arrow.

A. Brúzzi A. da S. (1962)

...the pulp...is poisonous....
[and] stupefies fish...

## An efficient fish poison of the Vaupés Indians

*Río Kuduyarí, Vaupés*

All of the Indians of the Colombian Vaupés use the leaves and crushed fruits of *Caryocar microcarpum* (and possibly other species of the Caryocaraceae) mixed and powdered with mud in holes in the ground. When fully mixed, the mud and vegetal remains are cast into pools as a fish poison. Whatever led primitive peoples to discover such a novel method of utilizing a toxic plant remains to be explained.

Recent work has shown that *Caryocar* contains triterpene saponins, a class of compounds known to be toxic to fish as well as to many insects. The leaves are known to be toxic to leaf-cutting ants.

...several species of plants are habitually employed and they differ greatly in the intensity of their toxicity to the fish. When large and deep pools are to be treated, the amount of poison introduced is very considerable, and the more active varieties of poisons are employed....

H.H. Rusby (1933)

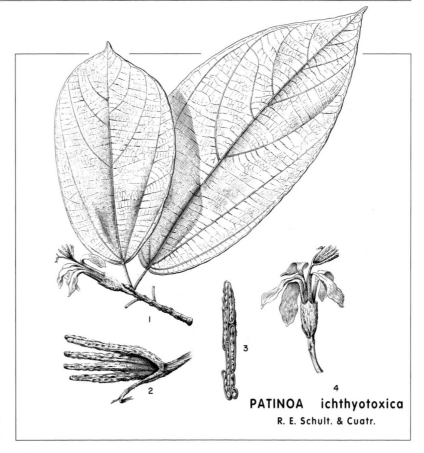

PATINOA ichthyotoxica
R. E. Schult. & Cuatr.

Several species...differ...
in their toxicity....

# A recently discovered minor fish poison

*Río Loretoyacu, Amazonas*

Every botanical expedition to the northwest Amazon seems to discover a new source of fish poisons. Recently, in the Loretoyacu River of Colombian Amazonas, a curious ichthyotoxic plant was discovered. It was a species new to science, *Patinoa ichthyotoxica* of the Bombacaceae or Kapok Family.

The Tikuna Indians of the area gather the pulp from the large fruit and dry it for use on short fishing expeditions. The seeds, roasted, are edible. The pulp, dried and powdered, is carried in pouches. It is cast into stagnant pools and within 20 minutes fish appear at the surface to obtain oxygen and are easily caught.

Nothing is known of the chemistry of this plant, but recent studies indicate the presence of alkaloids and phenolic substances in several members of the family.

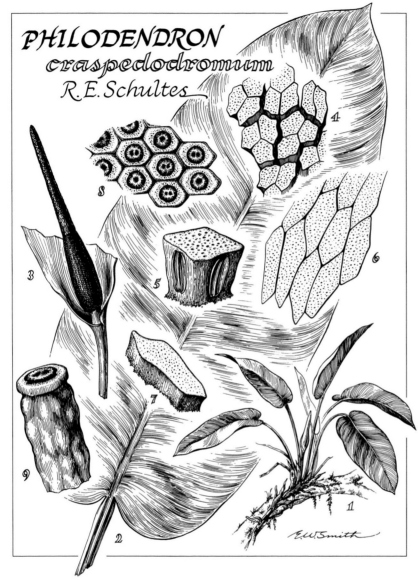

*PHILODENDRON craspedodromum R.E. Schultes*

Well over 100 different plants are on record as being used as piscicides by South American natives; this total is greater than that from any other continent.

R.F. Heizer (1949)

…over 100…plants… used as piscicides…

## An unusual fish poison

*Río Vaupés, Vaupés*

An unusual method of preparing fish poisons is common in the Colombian Vaupés. It involves cutting off the leaves and petioles of a large coriaceous aroid *(Philodendron craspedodromum)* and tying them tightly into small bundles. These are then set on the forest floor for several days to "steam" and start fermentation and rotting before being crushed and cast into stagnant water.

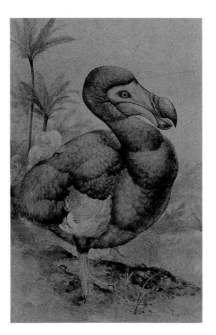

*Who knows what plants of
potential medical or other
value, quite apart from their
scientific interest, have already
gone the way of the dodo?*

R. Darnley Gibbs (1974)

# Epilogue

Natural healing has become one of the widely discussed topics of our time. Interest in the connection between the mind and body, how the food we eat affects our health, and the use of plants as medicines have never been greater. Tenets held sacred by natural physicians, long ignored by allopaths, are slowly but surely working their way into so-called "conventional" medicine.

Professors Schultes and Raffauf have taken us on a journey to a place where healing with plants is the norm, and where ritual and magic play an essential role in everyday life. Despite the fact that these pictures were taken several decades ago, in some of the areas depicted life remains remarkably similar, which is especially surprising in view of the outside forces working to drive the native cultures to extinction. In many cases, perhaps the outward appearance of the traditional healers, or payés as they are called in this region, has changed. However, their beliefs in spirits, in the value of plants as therapies and their use of ritual in healing ceremonies has not.

My first visit to this verdant ecosystem was in 1976, at the urging of Professor Schultes, who suggested that I "experience the Amazon." Travelling with then fellow graduate student Dr. James Zarucchi, we explored some of the same rivers that Schultes had visited 30 years before. We had the opportunity to work with several of his field assistants, or even their children, now old enough to strike out on their own into the forest. Sitting around the fire at night, we heard stories, now legends, of my mentor and friend. Tales were told of adventures that would send chills up our spines, as rapids tore boats apart, disease inflicted great adversity upon the scientists and their guides, airplanes were lost, or crucial provisions and equipment disappeared for unknown reasons. Back in Cambridge, with his characteristic modesty and good humour, Schultes would deny that anything out of the ordinary had happened, admonishing his students that anyone who searched for adventures in the field probably should not have been there in the first place. The record of this man's accomplishments is a phenomenal one, especially as it took place in an age when global travel was so difficult, and computers and other such technology only a dream. *Vine of the Soul* contains some of the most significant photographs on this subject ever taken, and it is a delight to know that this ethnobotanical information will be preserved and disseminated through the publication of this book.

Drs. Schultes and Raffauf have collaborated for many years as a multidisciplinary team, with Dr. Raffauf bringing his vast knowledge and perspectives as a plant chemist to numerous jointly authored papers and books. This latest collaboration brings together an extraordinary amount of information on the ethnobotany and phytochemistry of the plants used by the people of this region, and presents it in a way that is fascinating and inspiring to us all. In many ways, this book evokes memories of one of the most interesting courses I took in graduate school, taught by this team, "Plant Chemistry and Human Affairs." Only when disciplinary boundaries are crossed can scientists truly explore the full potential of a subject, reaching the most interesting and meaningful conclusions possible. This is the great achievement of Schultes and Raffauf in writing *Vine of the Soul*, and it will be appreciated as a classic work for many generations. I am honored and delighted to join my colleague Professor G.T. Prance in helping to launch this most significant book.

Michael J. Balick, F.L.S.
Director and Philecology
Curator of Economic Botany,
Institute of Economic Botany,
The New York Botanical Garden

# Glossary

achiote — a red dye-plant, *Bixa Orellana*.

alkaloid — a nitrogen-containing substance found in plants and some animals, often possessing a high degree of biological activity on other organisms and sometimes highly toxic.

ambíl — a tobacco preparation made by boiling the leaves with water and evaporating the solution to the consistency of honey.

anthropomorphic — having human shape or characteristics as applied to gods, animals or even inanimate objects.

ayahuasca — "vine of the soul" (*Banisteriopsis Caapi*).

barbasco — the general name among South American peoples for a plant used as a fish poison.

beta-carbolines — alkaloids which belong to a class of compounds known as MAO (monoamine oxidase) inhibitors which prevent normal metabolism of certain neurotransmitters, thus permitting their accumulation in the central nervous system. One result, for example, is the over-stimulation of brain functions dependent upon the transmitter serotonin which may manifest itself as hallucination.

blow gun — a long tube-like weapon through which darts or pellets are blown.

bodaquera — the Spanish term for blow gun.

Boraró — a kind of supernatural creature said to live in the forests.

borrachero — a term applied to many plants that cause intoxication.

caapi — a liana (*Banisteriopsis Caapi*) found in the Amazon forests and containing alkaloids capable of inducing hallucinations.

caatinga — in the northwest Amazonia the name given to isolated stretches of forests of slender trees on more or less xerophytic white sand and characterized usually by high endemism.

cacao — the proper name for the tree, source of chocolate, *Theobroma Cacao*. English-speaking people usually call it "cocoa".

cajuayá — a name given to several palms of the genus *Mauritiella*.

cananguche — the name in the Colombian Amazonia of *Mauritia minor* and *M. flexuosa*.

capitán — a word commonly applied to a payé, especially if he also serves as a civil leader.

cardiotonic — an agent having a tonic effect on the heart.

carurú — a name given to various members of the family Podostemonaceae, river weeds, extremely abundant in Amazonia.

cassava — the flour prepared from *Manihot esculenta* (manioc).

cerbatana — a Spanish term for blow gun.

chacruna — a local name for *Psychotria viridis* (Rubiaceae), an additive to caapi used widely in the western Amazon.

chagropanga — a local name for *Diplopterys Cabrerana* (Malpighiaceae) often added to the caapi drink.

chicha — a mildly alcoholic beverage prepared by fermentation of manioc, various fruits or sugar cane.

chiquichique — a name applied in the Colombian Amazon to the palm *Leopoldinia Piassaba*.

chiricaspi — *Brunfelsia Chiricaspi*.

chiric-sanango — *Brunfelsia grandiflora* var. *Schultesii*.

chivé — a watery porridge of manioc flour.

| | |
|---|---|
| *chontadura* | the vernacular name used throughout the Colombian Amazonia for the cultivated fruit palm *Guilielma speciosa*, known also as *Bactris Gasipaes*. |
| *chupé del tabaco* | a tobacco syrup used by sucking or licking or placing over the gums. |
| *coca* | the plant from which cocaine is isolated, *Erythroxylon Coca*. |
| *cocaine* | the most important of several alkaloids in the coca plant. It is a mild stimulant and acts also to assuage the feelings of hunger and fatigue. It is used in modern medicine as a local anesthetic in eye, ear, nose and throat surgery; its illicit use in non-Indian cultures is now common knowledge. |
| *cojamba* | the local name of Helosis in Amazonian Colombia. |
| *cola* | an African plant rich in caffeine, *Cola nitida*. |
| *comisaría* | a political division of Colombia in which the population is sparse. |
| *coumarin* | a white. crystalline, vanilla-flavoured substance obtained from several plants or prepared synthetically. |
| *cuchara-caspi* | the common name for a riparian plant, *Malouetia Tamaquarina*. |
| *culebra borrachero* | the local name in Sibundoy for the strong hallucinogen, *Methysticodendron Amesianum*. |
| *cunapurú* | in British Guiana, the name of a species of Phyllanthus used as a fish poison. |
| *curaca* | the name for a payé or medicine man in some parts of the Colombian Amazon. |
| *curandero* | a Spanish term for a medicine man. |
| *Curupira* | a monster living in the forests who waylays men by misleading them; see kurupira. |
| *cyanogenic glycosides* | compounds which liberate toxic cyanide on hydrolysis. These can be removed by boiling with water, discarding the liquid and squeezing out the remainder from the residual starchy root of manioc which is then suitable for consumption. |
| *da-pá-kö-da* | a plant (*Mandevilla Steyermarkii*) used as a medicinal panacea by the Kubeos. |
| *fariña* | the meal prepared from the tapioca plant. |
| *gahpi-ghori* | visions produced by the "vine of the soul". |
| *glycoside* | a compound containing a carbohydrate (sugar) as part of its chemical structure. |
| *guaraná* | a Brazilian caffeine-rich plant, *Paullinia Cupana*. |
| *guarumo* | any of many species of Cecropia, particularly (in connection with coca) the tall tree *C. sciadophylla*. |
| *guayuco* | the loin cloth worn by Indian men. |
| *guayusa* | the holly, *Ilex Guayusa*, the leaves of which are used to prepare a stimulating, caffeine-containing drink similar to our tea, sometimes spelled *huayusa*. |
| *hallucinogen* | a plant or other substance capable of producing the apparent perception of sights, sounds and tactility that are not actually present. |
| *hata* | a Venezuealan word for a long-flowering plant, the identification of which is unknown. |
| *igarapés* | channels or creeks of the major rivers. |
| *ipadú* | the Brazilian name of coca. |
| *jaguar* | an animal of the cat family found in Central and South America similar to the leopard but somewhat larger. |
| *Kai-ya-ree* | a four-day dance held at the time of |

the harvest of the peach palm, consisting of many individual masked dances beginning with one propitiating the forces of darkness and ending with the dance of the sun. The intervening dances are dedicated to many different animals and may be interpreted almost in an evolutionary sense.

*kana*    a rubiaceous plant with superstitious uses, *Sabicea amazonensis*.

*kinde borrachero*    one of the most atrophied clones of *Brugmansia aurea* in the Valley of Sibundoy.

*Kurupira*    see Boraró.

*liana*    a large woody vine.

*lingua geral*    a Tupi Indian language widely understood in many parts of the Brazilian Amazonia, officially called Nhengatí.

*llanos*    grasslands or plains in the Orinoco drainage of Colombia and Venezuela.

*mai-d'-agua*    "mother of waters" in Portugese; a faery who frequents rivers to enchant young couples with her singing.

*maloca*    a large communal house in which live several Indian families related by blood or marriage. It may be rectangular or circular, according to the tribe.

*ma-né-pa-ree-nee*    a medicinal plant used by the Taiwanos (*Bonnetia holostylis*).

*manguaré*    see tunday.

*manioc*    the cassava plant (*Manihot esculenta*) cultivated in the tropics for its large tuberous roots which contain much starch used as a basic food plant in large areas of South America. The starch is familiar to us as tapioca which is prepared therefrom.

*médico*    a doctor; the term is often employed to mean medicine man.

*mesetas*    the flat quartzitic mountains of Cretaceous age in the Colombian Amazonia.

*mingau*    a mixture of manioc and water, a kind of porridge.

*mirití*    a name for several species of palms of the genus Mauritia.

*munchiro borrachero*    one of the severely atrophied strains of the narcotic *Brugmansia aurea* in Sibundoy.

*Nyi*    goddess of the waters or rivers; a beautiful petroglyph on the Río Piraparaná.

*oco-yajé*    a Taiwano name for *Diplopterys Cabrerana*, a plant often used as a additive in the preparation of caapi.

*pajuíl*    *Nothocrax urumutum*, a partially domesticated and edible bird of the Amazon.

*payé*    a term used in Colombia and Ecuador for a medicine man or shaman.

*pedidya*    a flower worn as a love charm amongst the Kubeos.

*petroglyph*    a rock engraving.

*piassaba*    the fibre-yielding palm *Leopoldinia Piassaba*.

*purgative*    a substance capable of producing bowel movement; a cathartic.

*rotenone*    a compound found in certain plants used by native peoples as a fish poison and in commerce as an insecticide; it has a low toxicity for birds and mammals.

*saponins*    compounds which foam in water, behaving like soap. They are toxic to fish by reducing the surface tension at the gills, thereby preventing the uptake of oxygen from the water. Fish rise to the surface where the oxygen concentration is greater and are scooped up in nets or baskets.

*shaman*    a medicine man or payé.

*solimán*    (solymán) the rubiaceous plant *Duroia*

*hirsuta,* a mysterious plant with superstitious connections and valued as a fish poison.

steroid — any of a group of compounds containing a tetracyclic carbon skeleton related to cholesterol and certain animal hormones.

susto — a psychological fear of death or illness caused by certain hexes or other influences as a result of supernatural forces believed by the patient.

tepuí — the isolated, high, grotesquely eroded mountains in British Guiana and southern Venezuela.

tipitipi — a manioc squeezer.

tryptamines — indole alkyl amines, one of which is serotonin, a neuro-transmitter of the mammalian central nervous system. By delaying the deamination reactions in normal brain metabolism, tryptamines prolong the effects of serotonin in the body, one of which results in a hallucinatory state when the amount reaching the brain is sufficiently high.

d-tubocurarine — the active principle in Chondrodendron curares, which blocks the transmission of impulses from nerve to muscle, resulting in depression or paralysis of muscular activity.

tunday — a large drum used to communicate by sound through the forest.

Uaxti — type of supernatural creature supposed to inhabit the deep forests (Wagti).

Urubú-coará — an Indian house site on the Uaupés River, Brazil, near the Colombian frontier. The word means "vulture's nest".

uvilla — the name for a cultivated tree, *Pourouma cecropaeifolia,* source of a grape-like edible fruit. Its leaves may provide an ash to mix with coca powder.

Vai-mahsë — the supernatural Master of Animals.

viho — another name for the snuff prepared from various species of Virola. See also yakee.

Wagti — see Uaxti.

We-ra — a sacred Yukuna dance performed without uniforms; the traditional breech-cloth is worn.

wourali — the name for curare in the Guianas.

yajé — "vine of the soul" *(Banisteriopsis Caapi).*

yakee — the Puinave name for the snuff prepared from the powdered resin of various species of Virola.

yaupón — the name of the caffeine-rich shrub *Ilex vomitoria,* of south-eastern United States.

ye-cha — the Yukuna name of the tree *Micrandra Spruceana,* the seeds of which resemble anaconda eggs.

yerba maté — the caffeine-rich plant, *Ilex paraguariensis,* of Argentina and southern Brazil.

yoco — a vine *(Paullinia Yoco)* the bark of which is the source of a caffeine-containing stimulating drink.

yoco blanco — one of the kinds of the yoco vine recognized by the Indians.

yoco colorado — one of the most abundant kinds of *Paullinia Yoco.*

yopo — a narcotic snuff prepared from the seeds of *Anadenanthera peregrina.*

yuca — the plant from which manioc and tapioca are prepared *(Manihot esculenta);* also the flour prepared from it.

Yuruparí — (Brazilian = jurupari) a dance in which only the males who blow sacred bark trumpets participate and which may be part of a cult of ancestral worship, an initiation ceremony, or sometimes, a dedication to malevolent demons.

Agassiz, Prof. Louis and Mrs. Elizabeth Cary. *A Journey in Brazil*. Ticnor and Fields, Boston (1868).

Allen, P.H. Indians of Southeastern Colombia. Geographical Review 37 (1947) 567-582.

Barco, V., President of Colombia, in a speech to the Witoto Indians in La Chorrera, Rio Igaraparaná, April, 1988.

Baudelaire, C. *Artificial Paradises*. Transl. by E. Fox. Herder and Herder, New York (1971).

Bown, D. *Aroids: Plants of the Arum Family*. Timber Press, Portland, Oregon (1988).

Brüzzi-A., A da S. *A Civilicaõ Indígena do Uaupés*. Linográfica Editora, Ltda., São Paulo (1962).

Cutright, P. *The Great Naturalists Explore South America*. MacMillan Co., London (1940).

Dobkin de Rios, M. Curing with ayahuasca in urban slums. In M.J. Harner, *Hallucinogens and Shamanism*. Oxford University Press, New York (1973).

Dominguez, C.A. In D. Samper, *Naturaleza y Cultura Amazónica del Bajo Caquetá*. Instituto de Ciéncias Naturales, Bogotá (1987) 31-54.

Emboden, W. *Narcotic Plants*. MacMillan Pub. Co. New York, (Ed. 2) (1979).

Franciscan Report on Missionary Activity along the Rio Putumayo (1773). See Patiño (1967).

García-Barriga, H. *Flora Medicinal de Colombia*. Instituto de Ciéncias Naturales, Bogotá 1 (1974).

Gibbs, R.D. *Chemotaxonomy of Flowering Plants*. McGill-Queens University Press, Montreal (1974).

Gill. R. *White Water and Black Magic*. Henry Holt and Co., New York (1940).

Goldman, I. Tribes of the Uaupés-Caquetá region. In J.H. Steward (Ed.), *Handbook of the South American Indians*. U.S. Govt. Printing Office, Washington, D.C. 3 (1948).

————*The Cubeo: Indians of the Northwest Amazon*. Illinois Studies Anthropology, Urbana, Illinois, N. 2 (1960).

Hardenburg, W.E. *The Putumayo: The Devil's Paradise*. T. Fisher Unwin, London (1912).

Harner, M.J. (Ed.). *Hallucinogens and Shamanism*. Oxford University Press, New York (1973).

Hegnauer, R. *Chemotaxonomie der Pflanzen*. Birkhäuser Verlag, Basel, Vols. 1-7 (1962-1986).

Heizer, R.F. Fish poisons. In J.H. Steward (Ed.), *Handbook of the South American Indians*. U.S. Govt. Printing Office, Washington, D.C. 5 (1949).

Heywood, V.H., *et al*. *Flowering Plants of the World*. Mayflower Books, New York (1978).

*Holy Bible*. Revised Berkeley Version, Gideon International, Nashville, Tennessee (1976).

Hudson. W.H. *Green Mansions*. Heritage Press. New York (1936).

Hugh-Jones, S. *The Palm and the Pleiades: Initiation and Chronology in Northwest Amazonia*. Cambridge Univ. Press, Cambridge, England (1979).

Imthurn, E.F. *Among the Indians of Guiana*. K. Paul, Trench and Co., London (1883).

Jiménez de Espada, M. (1738). In Patiño, M. Econ. Bot. 22 (1968) 311-316.

Kamen-Kaye, D. Chimo — an unusual form of tobacco in Venezuela. Bot. Mus. Leaflets, Harvard Univ. 23 (1971) 35.

Koch-Grünberg, T. *Südamerikanische Felszeichnungen*. Ernst Wasmuth, Berlin (1907).

————*Zwei Jahre unter den Indianern*. Ernst Wasmuth, Berlin, Vol. I (1909), Vol. II (1910).

Kostermans, A.J., H.V. Pinkley and W.L. Stern. A new Amazonian arrow poison: *Ocotea venenosa*. Bot Mus. Leaflets, Harvard Univ. 22 (1969) 241-252.

LaBarre, W. Hallucinogens and the shamanistic origins of religion. In P.T. Furst, *Flesh of the Gods*. Praeger Publishers, New York (1972).

Lamb, F.B. *Rio Tigre and Beyond. The Amazon Jungle Medicine of Manuel Cordova*. North Atlantic Books, Berkeley (1985).

LaRotta, C. *Observaciones Etnobotánicas sobre Algunas Especies Utilizadas por la Comunidad Indígena Andoque (Amazonas Colombia)*. Corporación de Araracuara, Bogotá (1983).

Le Cointe, P. *Amazonia Brasileira III. Arvores e Plantas Uteis*. Livraria Classica, Belém do Pará, Brazil (1934).

Levi-Strauss. The use of wild plants in tropical South America. In J.H. Steward (Ed.), *Handbook of South American Indians*. U.S. Govt. Printing Office, Washington D.C. 6 (1950) 465-486.

Lewin. L. *Die Pfeilgifte*. Verlag von Johann Ambrosius Barth. Leipzig (1923); Reprinted, Verlag Gerstenberg, Hildesheim (1971).

Lewin, L. *Phantastica: Narcotic and Stimulating Drugs*. Kegan Paul, Trench Truebener and Co., Ltd. London (1931). Reprinted, Routledge and Kegan Paul, London (1964).

Lewis, W.H. and M.P.F. Lewis. *Medical Botany. Plants Affecting Man's Health*. John Wiley and Sons, New York (1977).

Lockwood, T.E. The ethnobotany of *Brugmansia*. Journ. Ethnopharmacol. 1 (1979) 147-164.

Lowie, R.H. The tropical forest tribes. In J.H. Steward (Ed.). *Handbook of South American Indians*. U.S. Govt. Printing Office, Washington, D.C. 3 (1948).

Mac Creagh, G. *White Waters and Black*. Century Co., New York (1926).

Mariani-Ramírez, C. *Temas de Hipnosis*. Editorial Andres Bello, Santiago de Chile (1965) 362-363, t.23.

Martin, R.T. The role of coca in history, religion and medicine of South American Indians. Econ. Bot. 24 (1970) 422-438.

McGovern, W.M. *Jungle Paths and Inca Ruins*. The Century Co., New York (1927).

McKenna, D.J., L.E. Luna and G.H.N. Powers. Biodynamic constituents in Ayahuasca admixture plants: an uninvestigated folk pharmacopoeia. America Indígena 46 (1986) 73.

McKenna. T. Plan, plant, planet. Whole Earth. No. 64 (1989) 10.

Meggers. B.J. *Amazonia. Man and Culture in a Counterfeit Paradise*. Aldine-Atherton. Inc., Chicago (1971).

Métraux, A. Weapons. In J.H. Steward (Ed.) *Handbook of South American Indians*. U.S. Govt. Printing Office, Washington, D.C. 5 (1949) 229-263.

Monardes, N. *Joyfull Newes Out of the Newe Founde Worlde* (1574). Transl. by John Frampton. Constable and Co., Ltd., London; A.A. Knopf, New York (1925).

Mortimer, W.G. *History of Coca, The Divine Plant of the Incas* J.H. Vail and Co., New York (1901).

Moser, B. and D. Tayler. *The Cocaine Eaters*. Longmans, London (1965).

Nery, Baron de. See Santa-Ana.

Pagan, Count. Transl. by William Hamilton. *An Historical and Geographical Description of the Great County and River of the Amazones in America*. John Starkey, London (1663).

Patiño, V.M. *Plantas Cultivadas y Animales Domésticos en Amazonia Equinoccial. Vol 3, Fibras, Medicinas, Miscellaneas*. Imprenta Departmental, Cali Vol. 3 (1967) 259.

Pérez-Arbeláez, E. In D. Bovet-Nitti and G.B. Marini-Bettolo (Eds.). *Curare and Curare-like Agents*. Elsevier Publ. Co., Amsterdam (1959).

Plotkin, M. Personal Communication. Lecture, Harvard University, April 1985.

Plowman, T. Folk uses of New World aroids. Econ. Bot. 23 (1969) 115.

————Four new Brunfelsias from northwestern South America. Bot. Mus. Leaflets, Harvard Univ. 23 (1973) 245-272.

———— Brunfelsia in ethnomedicine. Bot. Mus. Leaflets, Harvard Univ. 25 (1977) 289-320.

———— Amazonian coca. Journ. Ethnopharmacol. 3 (1981) 195-225.

Radin, P. *Indians of South America*. Doubleday, Doran and Co., Garden City, N.Y. (1942).

Ralegh, Sir Walter. In R. Schomburgk: *Ralegh's Discovery of Guiana*. Hakluyt Society, London (1848).

Readers Digest Association. *Health Guide and Medical Encyclopedia* 1970.

Reichel-Dolmatoff, G. *Desana. Simbolísmo de los Indios Tukanos del Vaupés*. Universidad de los Andes, Bogotá (1968).

————*Amazonian Cosmos: the Sexual and Religious Symbolism of the Tukano Indians*. Univ. of Chicago Press, Chicago (1971).

———— The cultural context of an aboriginal halluci-nogen—*Banisteriopsis Caapi*. In P.T. Furst, *Flesh of the Gods*. Praeger Publishers, New York (1972).

———— *The Shaman and the Jaguar. A Study of Narcotic Drugs among the Indians of Colombia*. Temple Univ. Press, Philadelphia (1975).

———— In Litt. (1990).

Rheingold, H. Ethnobotany and the search for van-ishing knowledge. Whole Earth No. 64 (1989) 16-23.

Robinson, S.S. *Toward an Understanding of Kofán Sha-manism*. Latin American Studies Program, Disser-tation Series, Cornell University, No. 74 (1979).

Roth, W.E. An introductory study of the arts, crafts and customs of the Guiana Indians. 38th Ann. Rept. Bur. Amer. Ethnol. 1916-1917. Washington, D.C. (1924).

Rouse, I. Petroglyphs. In J.H. Steward (Ed.). *Handbook of South American Indians*. U.S. Govt. Printing Of-fice, Washington, D.C. 5 (1949) 493-502.

Rusby, H.H. *Jungle Memories*. Whittlesey House, McGraw Hill Book Co., New York (1933).

Santa-Ana Nery, Baron of. Transl. by G. Humphery. *The Land of the Amazons*. Sands and Co., London (1901).

Schery, R.W. *Plants for Man*. Prentice Hall Inc., Englewood Cliffs, New Jersey (Ed. 2.)(1972).

Seeman, B. *Popular History of the Palms and Their Allies*. Lovell, Reeve, London (1856).

Seitz, G.J. In D.H. Efron, B. Holmstedt and N.S. Kline (Eds.). *Ethnopharmacologic Search for Psychoactive Drugs*. U.S. Govt. Printing Office (1967). Reprinted, Raven Press, New York (1979).

Sharon, D. The San Pedro cactus in Peruvian folk healing. In P.T. Furst, *Flesh of the Gods*. Praeger, New York (1972) 114-135.

Shemluck, M. The flowers of *Ilex Guayusa*. Bot. Mus. Leaflets, Harvard Univ. 27 (1979) 155-160.

———— Ph.D. Thesis, Northeastern Univ., Boston, Mass. J. Nat. Prod. 54 (1991) 1601-1606.

Simson, A. Notes on the Piajes of the Putumayo. Royal Journ. Anthrop. Inst. Gr. Brit. and Ireland. 3 (1879) 213.

Spruce, R. Geographical Magazine (c.1870). Reprinted in (A.R. Wallace, Ed.) *Notes of a Botanist on the Amazon and Andes*. MacMillan and Co, London, 2 (1908) 453, and by Johnson Reprint Corp., New York 2 (1970).

Steward, J.H. and H. Métraux. The Tropical Forest Tribes. In J.H. Steward (Ed.). *Handbook of South American Indians*. U.S. Govt. Printing Office, Wash-ington, D.C. 3 (1948) 605.

Stone, D. In J.H. Steward (Ed.). *Handbook of South American Indians*. U.S. Govt. Printing Office, Wash-ington, D.C. 4 (1948) 215.

Thielkuhl, J.F. Introducción al estudio del *Methysticondendron Amesianum*. Universidad Nacional, Bogotá (1957). Thesis, in ed.

Trupp, F. *The Last Indians: South American's Cultural Heritage*. Perlinger Verlag, Wörgl, Austria (1981).

Uphof, J.C.T. *Dictionary of Economic Plants*. Verlag J. Cramer, Lehre, Germany (1968).

Von Martius, C.F.P. See Von Spix, J.B.

Von Spix, J.B. and C.F.P. von Martius. *Travels in Brazil in the Years 1817-1820*. Longman, Hurst, Rees, Orme, Brown and Green (1824).

Walton, J.W. Muinane diagnostic use of narcotics. Econ. Bot. 24 (1970) 187-188.

Waterton, C. *Wanderings in South America* (1825), Sturgis and Walton Co. New York (1909).

Watt, J.M. Magic and witchcraft in relation to plants and folk medicine. In T. Swain (Ed.). *Plants in the Development of Modern Medicine*. Harvard Univ. Press, Cambridge, Mass. (1972) 67-102.

Whiffen, T. *The Northwest Amazon. Notes on Some Months Spent among the Cannibal Tribes*. Constable and Co., London (1915).

Wilbert, J. *Tobacco and Shamanism in South America*. Yale Univ. Press, New Haven, Conn. (1987).

Zerda-Bayón, R. *Informe del Jefe de la Expedición Científica del Año de 1905 a 1906*, Bogotá (1906).

# Where the Gods Reign
## *Plants and Peoples*
## *of the Colombian Amazon*

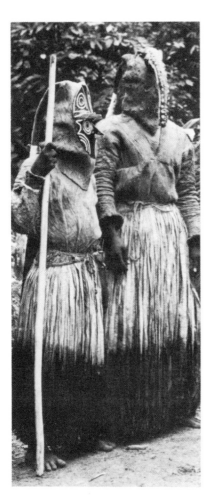

**By Richard Evans Schultes,**
Director (Emeritus),
Harvard Botanical Museum

This is a major work in the field of ethnobotany—the study of the various uses of plants by indigenous cultures. The author is one of the great Amazonian explorers of this century. The knowledgeable text is enhanced by 140 black and white photographs taken during the period of his travels between 1940 and 1954. Prince Philip presented Dr. Schultes with the World Wildlife Fund Gold Medal in 1984, calling him "the father of ethnobotany".

*Where the Gods Reign* offers the opportunity to journey the mysterious Colombian Amazon with this most remarkable scientist and eloquent guide. The Introduction includes a concise overview to the Amazon in general, followed by description of the Colombian Amazon where Dr. Schultes spent the majority of these fourteen years in the field living and studying the people and their plants.

The Indian people who possess the knowledge gathered over many generations of the effects of various plants on the human body and psyche, have unique insights into the deeper levels of ecology. They still understand the properties of some plants which western science has yet to assimilate. But, the way of life which supports this wealth of knowledge is fast disappearing. This makes Schultes' book all the more important, as is its sequel *Vine of the Soul: Medicine Men, Their Plants and Rituals in the Colombian Amazon.*

"Richard Schultes is a true ethno-botanist, the incarnation and almost the inventor of this discipline… *Where the Gods Reign* is a picture book, …of great beauty and tranquility …full of fascinating information."

– Sir John Hemming,
*Times Literary Supplement*

"*Where the Gods Reign* is a magnificent book by one of the greatest Amazon explorers of this century —a must for the library of any Amazon oriented person."

– Dr. Ghillean Prance,
Royal Botanic Gardens, Kew

"The numerous photographs are at once spectacular, beautiful, fascinating, and of excellent quality … It is likely that only Professor Schultes has had or ever will have the resources to produce such… a remarkable book."

– Willard Van Adsall,
*Journal of Ethnobiology*

$20 paperback, 312 pgs., ISBN 0 907791 131

Synergetic Press

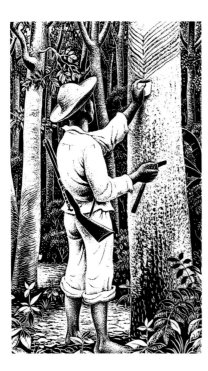

# White Gold:
# The Diary of a Rubber Cutter
# in the Amazon 1906-1916

**By John C. Yungjohann**
**Edited by Ghillean T. Prance**

The crisis of the rainforest began a century ago when it was discovered to be a source of rubber. This brought commercial interests into collision with this complex ecology—its plants, its animals and its peoples. At the height of the rubber boom in the early years of this century, a young American, John Yungjoham, struggled for survival as a rubber cutter. The diaries he kept have recently come to light and have been edited by Ghillean Prance of the Royal Botanic Gardens at Kew, England, one of the foremost botanical gardens in the world. Dr. Prance is a leading expert on the rainforest.

The diaries are especially poignant since the rubber cutters of today are fighting to preserve the forest against the ravages of the indiscriminate destruction which still ignores the true wealth of the region—its almost incomprehensible variety of species. It is a tale of humanity and the natural order working together in the midst of greed and ignorance. Ghillean Prance enhances the text with his own contemporary photographs and identifies the fungi, plants and animals which are mentioned in the pages of the diaries.

"Readers of this journal will find this first hand account fascinating and will appreciate the efforts of a work weary rubber cutter to not only survive the experience but to write about it."

– *Journal of Ethnobiology*

"How fortunate that the diary of the American youth John Yungjohann has come to light and that the famous botanist Dr. Ghillean Prance, with years of experience in the Amazon, has so understandably edited it."

– Dr. Richard Evans Schultes, Director (Emeritus), Harvard Botanical Museum

"It is thoroughly pleasing, easy reading, and would make a good supplement to a high school or college course that deals with economic plants or the Amazon… Plan on reading it in one sitting."

– George K. Rogers, Missouri Botanical Garden

$7.95 paperback, 104 pgs.,  ISBN 0 907791 166

Synergetic Press